Mind Maps
for Medical
Students

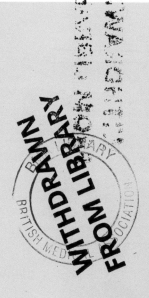

22/6/11
21/02/201

Mind Maps for Medical Students

Olivia Smith

The Hull York Medical School, UK

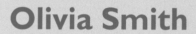

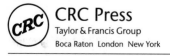

CRC Press
Taylor & Francis Group
Boca Raton London New York

CRC Press is an imprint of the
Taylor & Francis Group, an **informa** business

CRC Press
Taylor & Francis Group
6000 Broken Sound Parkway NW, Suite 300
Boca Raton, FL 33487-2742

© 2015 by Taylor & Francis Group, LLC
CRC Press is an imprint of Taylor & Francis Group, an Informa business

No claim to original U.S. Government works

Printed on acid-free paper
Version Date: 20141104

International Standard Book Number-13: 978-1-4822-5031-2 (Paperback)

Visit the Taylor & Francis Web site at
http://www.taylorandfrancis.com

and the CRC Press Web site at
http://www.crcpress.com

Printed by Bell & Bain Ltd, Glasgow

Contents

In memory of Michael J. Webb

It would be wrong for me not to acknowledge the man to whom this book is dedicated. I know that without Michael's care and tireless patience I would never have undertaken, nor believed that I could complete, a project such as this.

Mind Maps for Medical Students represents an industrious and valuable piece of work from an undergraduate student. But perhaps I should start by saying what it is not. It is neither a textbook nor a definitive information source for students encountering a topic for the first time. It cannot give a comprehensive account of every topic listed and some information will change as the world of medicine rapidly evolves.

So what does *Mind Maps for Medical Students* offer? The author has provided rapid revision notes covering a broad range of medical topics, ideally suited to students and early postgraduates revising for exams. This distillation of knowledge will save many hours of note taking for other students. The format will appeal to those who construct their knowledge in logical sequences and the layout will allow the reader to add notes and annotations as information changes or to add a local context.

The author is to be congratulated on providing so much information in such a concise format and I hope that many others will be rewarded by her endeavours.

Colin H. Jones
MBChB, MD, FRCP, Master of Education
Associate Dean of Assessment, The Hull York Medical School, UK

I am extremely grateful to Dr. A.G.W. Smith and Dr. D. Maleknasr for their continued support, help and guidance with this project.

The idea for this book began when I was in my second year of medical school. It was only then that I truly realised the full enormity of knowledge that medical students have to retain.

I envisaged a book presenting relevant material in a simplified way that would only enhance and consolidate what I had already learned from textbooks, lectures and the ward, particularly in the countdown to exams. Then, as chance would have it, I was granted the opportunity to make this a reality.

This book is an attempt to cover the main topics faced by medical students from day one, capturing and presenting the facts in a clear manner that is even sufficient for final year level. Even its format has been designed with the student in mind – it is pocket sized and has titles covering the definition of the disease, causes, investigations, treatments and complications to aid recall. The intention of *Mind Maps for Medical Students* is not to substitute for larger texts but to complement them and, with that in mind, I hope that it assists your understanding.

Finally, I hope that readers enjoy this book and I wish you all the best of luck with your medical and future studies.

Olivia Smith
Fourth year medical student, The Hull York Medical School, UK

Abbreviations

5-ASA — 5-aminosalicylic acid
ABG — arterial blood gas
ACE — angiotensin converting enzyme
ACE-III — Addenbrooke's Cognitive Examination
ACTH — adrenocorticotrophic hormone
ADH — antidiuretic hormone
ADL — activity of daily living
ADP — adenosine diphosphate
ADPKD — autosomal dominant polycystic kidney disease
AF — atrial fibrillation
Ag — antigen
AIDS — acquired immunodeficiency syndrome
AKI — acute kidney injury
ALL — acute lymphoblastic leukaemia
AML — acute myeloid leukaemia
ANA — antinuclear antibody
ANCA — antineutrophil cytoplasmic antibody
APML — acute promyelocytic leukaemia
Apo — apolipoprotein
APP — amyloid precursor protein
ARB — angiotensin receptor blocker
ARDS — acute respiratory distress syndrome
ARPKD — autosomal recessive polycystic kidney disease
ASD — atrial septal defect
ATP — adenosine triphosphate
AV — atrioventricular
BBB — blood–brain barrier
BMI — body mass index
BNP — brain natriuretic peptide
BP — blood pressure

BPH — benign prostatic hypertrophy
CABG — coronary artery bypass graft
CADASIL — cerebral autosomal dominant arteriopathy with subcortical infarcts and leucoencephalopathy
CCP — cyclic citrullinated peptide
CEA — carcinoembryonic antigen
CHF — congestive heart failure
CJD — Creutzfeldt–Jakob disease
CKI — chronic kidney injury
CLL — chronic lymphocytic leukaemia
CML — chronic myeloid leukaemia
CMV — cytomegalovirus
CNS — central nervous system
COPD — chronic obstructive pulmonary disease
CRC — colorectal cancer
CRP — C-reactive protein
CSF — cerebrospinal fluid
CT — computed tomography
CTS — carpal tunnel syndrome
CXR — chest X-ray
DaTSCAN — ioflupane ^{123}I for injection
DCIS — ductal carcinoma in situ
DEXA — dual-energy X-ray scan
DFA — direct fluorescent antibody test
DHT — dihydrotestosterone
DI — diabetes insipidus
DIC — disseminated intravascular coagulation
DIP — distal interphalangeal (joint)
DM — diabetes mellitus
DMARD — disease modifying antirheumatic drug
DNA — deoxyribonucleic acid
DPP — dipeptidyl peptidase

DVLA	Driver and Vehicle Licensing Agency	**GLP**	glucagon-like peptide
DVT	deep vein thrombosis	**GnRH**	gonadotrophin releasing hormone
DWI	diffusion-weighted MRI	**GORD**	gastro-oesophageal reflux disease
EBV	Epstein–Barr virus	**Gp**	glycoprotein
ECG	electrocardiography	**GTN**	glyceryl trinitrate
ECHO	echocardiography	**HAART**	highly active antiretroviral therapy
EEG	electroencephalography	**HAV**	hepatitis A virus
EIA	enzyme immunoassay	**Hb**	haemoglobin
ELISA	enzyme linked immunosorbent assay	**HbAlc**	glycated haemoglobin
EMB	eosin methylene blue	**HBV**	hepatitis B virus
EMG	electromyography	**HCC**	hepatocellular carcinoma
EPEC	enteropathogenic *E. coli*	**HCV**	hepatitis C virus
EPO	erythropoietin	**HDV**	hepatitis D virus
ERCP	endoscopic retrograde cholangiopancreatography	**HEV**	hepatitis E virus
ESKD	end-stage kidney disease	**HGPRT**	hypoxanthine–guanine phosphoribosyltransferase
ESR	erythrocyte sedimentation rate	**HHV**	human herpes virus
ESWL	extracorporeal shock wave lithotripsy	**HIV**	human immunodeficiency virus
FAP	familial adenomatous polyposis	**HNPCC**	hereditary nonpolyposis colorectal cancer
FBC	full blood count	**HPV**	human papilloma virus
FEV1	forced expiratory volume	**HTLV-1**	human T-lymphotrophic virus-1
FSH	follicle stimulating hormone	**HUS**	haemolytic uraemic syndrome
FTA	fluorescent treponemal antibody absorption	**IBD**	inflammatory bowel disease
FVC	forced vital capacity	**IBS**	irritable bowel syndrome
GABA	gamma-amino butyric acid	**ICU**	intensive care unit
GBM	glomerular basement membrane	**IFA**	immunofluorescence assay
(c)GFR	(calculated) glomerular filtration rate	**Ig**	immunoglobulin
		IGF	insulin-like growth factor
GH	growth hormone	**IL**	interleukin
GHRH	growth hormone releasing hormone	**IOP**	intraocular pressure
		IPSS	International Prostate Symptom Score
GI	gastrointestinal	**IV**	intravenous
GIT	gastrointestinal tract	**IVU**	intravenous urogram
		JVP	jugular venous pressure

KUB	kidney, ureter, bladder	**NRTI**	nucleoside reverse transcriptase inhibitor
LBBB	left bundle branch block		
LFTs	liver function tests	**NSAID**	nonsteroidal anti-inflammatory drug
LH	luteinising hormone		
LHRH	luteinising hormone-releasing hormone	**NSCC**	non small cell carcinoma
		NSTEMI	non-ST elevation myocardial infarction
LMN	lower motor neuron		
LMWH	low molecular weight heparin	**OA**	osteoarthritis
LP	lumbar puncture	**PaCO$_2$**	arterial partial pressure of carbon dioxide
LTOT	long-term oxygen therapy		
LVF	left ventricular failure	**PaO$_2$**	arterial partial pressure of oxygen
MALT	mucosa-associated lymphoid tissue (lymphoma)		
		PAH	phenylalanine hydroxylase
MAO	monoamine oxidase	**PCI**	percutaneous coronary intervention
MCH	mean corpuscular haemoglobin		
		PCR	polymerase chain reaction
MCPJ	metacarpophalangeal joint	**PE**	pulmonary embolus
MCV	mean corpuscular volume	**PET**	positron emission tomography
MEN	multiple endocrine neoplasia (syndrome)	**PG**	prostaglandin
		PI	protease inhibitor
MI	myocardial infarction	**PIP**	proximal interphalangeal
MLCK	myosin light chain kinase	**PPAR**	peroxisome proliferator-activated receptor
MMR	mumps, measles, rubella		
MND	motor neuron disease		
MOA	mode of action	**PPI**	proton pump inhibitor
MRCP	magnetic resonance cholangiopancreatography	**PR**	per rectum
		PSA	prostate specific antigen
MRI	magnetic resonance imaging	**PT**	prothrombin time
MS	multiple sclerosis	**PTH**	parathyroid hormone
MTPJ	metatarsophalangeal joint	**PTT**	partial thromboplastin time
NAAT	nucleic acid amplification test	**RA**	rheumatoid arthritis
NBM	nil by mouth	**RAAS**	renin angiotensin aldosterone system
NICE	National Institute for Health and Care Excellence		
		RCC	renal cell carcinoma
NIV	noninvasive ventilation	**RDS**	respiratory distress syndrome
NMDA	N-methyl-D-aspartate	**RNA**	ribonucleic acid
NNRTI	non-nucleoside reverse transcriptase inhibitor	**RPR**	rapid plasma regain
		RVF	right ventricular failure
NPI	Nottingham Prognostic Index	**SCC**	small cell carcinoma
		SERM	selective oestrogen receptor modulator

SLE	systemic lupus erythematosus	**TOF**	tetralogy of Fallot
SPECT	single photon emission computed tomography	**TPHA**	*Treponema pallidum* haemagglutination test
SSRI	selective serotonin reuptake inhibitor	**TPPA**	*Treponema pallidum* particle agglutination test
STEMI	ST elevation myocardial infarction	**TSH**	thyroid stimulating hormone
STI	sexually transmitted infection	**TURP**	transurethral resection of the prostate
SUDEP	sudden unexplained death in epilepsy	**U&Es**	urine and electrolytes
T3	triiodothyronine	**UMN**	upper motor neuron
T4	thyroxine	**UPEC**	uropathogenic *E. coli*
TB	tuberculosis	**UTI**	urinary tract infection
TCC	transitional cell carcinoma	**VDRL**	Venereal Disease Research Laboratory
TFTs	thyroid function tests	**V/Q**	ventilation/perfusion
Th	T helper (cell)	**VSD**	ventricular septal defect
TIA	transient ischaemic attack	**VWF**	von Willebrand factor
TIBC	total iron binding capacity	**VZV**	varicella zoster virus
TNF	tumour necrosis factor	**WCC**	white cell count

Chapter One The Cardiovascular System

The Cardiovascular System

Map 1.1 Heart Failure

What is heart failure?

This may be defined as the inability of cardiac output to meet the physiological demands of the body. It can be classified in several ways:

- Left ventricular failure (LVF): Symptoms of LVF: paroxysmal nocturnal dyspnoea, wheeze, nocturnal cough with pink sputum caused by pulmonary oedema.
- Right ventricular failure (RVF): Symptoms of RVF, which is usually caused by LVF or lung disease, peripheral oedema and ascites.
- Low output and high output heart failure. This is due to excessive afterload, excessive preload or pump failure.

Pathophysiology

See page 4.

Causes

Anything that causes myocardial damage may lead to heart failure.
Examples include:

- Coronary artery disease.
- Hypertension.
- Atrial fibrillation.
- Valve disease.
- Cardiomyopathies.
- Infective endocarditis.
- Anaemia.
- Endocrine disorders.
- Cor pulmonale: this is right ventricular failure secondary to pulmonary disease.

Classification

Framingham Criteria for Congestive Heart Failure: 2 major criteria *or* 1 major criteria and 2 minor criteria:

- Major criteria: **PAINS**
  ○ Paroxysmal nocturnal dyspnoea.
  ○ Acute pulmonary oedema.
  ○ Increased heart size, Increased central venous pressure.
  Neck vein dilation.
  ○ S3 gallop.
- Minor criteria: **PAIN**
  ○ Pleural effusion.
  ○ Ankle oedema (bilateral).
  ○ Increased heart rate >120 beats/min.
  ○ Nocturnal cough.

New York Heart Association Classification for Heart Failure

I: No limitation of physical activity.
II: Slight limitation of physical activity.
III: Marked limitation of physical activity.
IV: Inability to carry out physical activity.

MAP 1.1 **Heart Failure**

Treatment

- Conservative: smoking cessation advice, weight loss, promotion of healthy diet and exercise.
- Medical:
  - **Angiotensin** converting enzyme (ACE) inhibitors.
  - **Beta-blockers**: currently only two are licensed in the UK, bisoprolol and carvedilol
  - **Candesartan**: an angiotensin receptor blocker (if intolerant to ACE inhibitors).
  - **Digoxin**: a cardiac glycoside.
  - **Diuretics**, e.g. furosemide.
  - **Spironolactone**: an aldosterone receptor antagonist.
- Surgical: heart transplantation.

Complications

- Renal failure.
- Valve dysfunction.
- Stroke.

Investigations

- Bloods:
  - FBC, U&Es, LFTs, TFTs, lipid profile.
  - BNP (brain natriuretic peptide).
    It suggests how much the myocytes are stretched. BNP is arguably cardioprotective as it causes Na^+ ion and H_2O excretion in addition to vasodilation. A concentration >400 pg/mL (>116 pmol/L) is suggestive of heart failure.
- CXR: **ABCDE**
  - **A**lveolar oedema.
  - Kerley **B** lines.
  - **C**ardiomegaly.
  - **D**ilated upper lobe vessels.
  - pleural **E**ffusion.
- ECHO: aims to identify cause and assess function of the heart.
- ECG.

Map 1.1 Heart Failure

The Cardiovascular System

Map 1.2 Pathophysiology of Congestive Heart Failure (CHF)

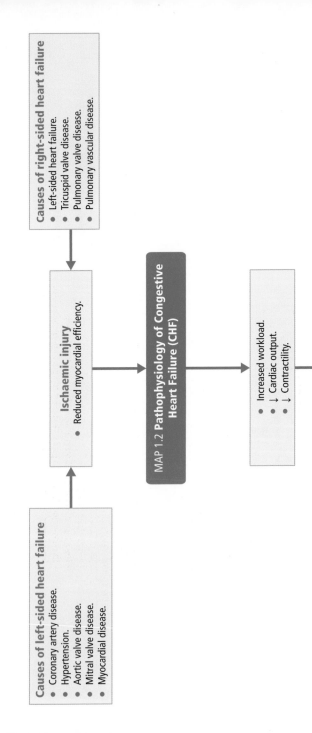

Causes of right-sided heart failure
- Left-sided heart failure.
- Tricuspid valve disease.
- Pulmonary valve disease.
- Pulmonary vascular disease.

Causes of left-sided heart failure
- Coronary artery disease.
- Hypertension.
- Aortic valve disease.
- Mitral valve disease.
- Myocardial disease.

Ischaemic injury
- Reduced myocardial efficiency.

MAP 1.2 Pathophysiology of Congestive Heart Failure (CHF)

- Increased workload.
- ↓ Cardiac output.
- ↓ Contractility.

Activates compensatory mechanisms

- Activation of the renin angiotensin aldosterone system (RAAS) causes Na^+ ion and H_2O retention, and peripheral vasoconstriction. This increases preload.
- Activation of the sympathetic nervous system increases heart rate and causes peripheral vasoconstriction. This increases afterload.
- ↑ Myocyte size.

Chronic activation of these compensatory mechanisms worsens heart failure and leads to increased cardiac damage.

Remember that:

- The cause of cardiac dilation is increased end-diastolic volume.
- The raised jugular venous pressure (JVP) is related to right-sided heart failure and fluid overload.
- Hepatomegaly is caused by congestion of the hepatic portal circulation.

Map 1.3 Myocardial Infarction (MI)

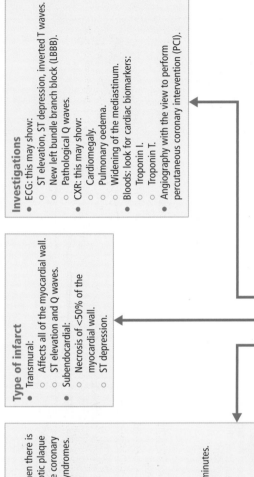

Investigations
- ECG: this may show:
  - ST elevation, ST depression, inverted T waves.
  - New left bundle branch block (LBBB).
  - Pathological Q waves.
- CXR: this may show:
  - Cardiomegaly.
  - Pulmonary oedema.
  - Widening of the mediastinum.
- Bloods: look for cardiac biomarkers:
  - Troponin I.
  - Troponin T.
- Angiography with the view to perform percutaneous coronary intervention (PCI).

Type of infarct
- Transmural:
  - Affects all of the myocardial wall.
  - ST elevation and Q waves.
- Subendocardial:
  - Necrosis of <50% of the myocardial wall.
  - ST depression.

MAP 1.3
Myocardial Infarction (MI)

What is MI?
Also known as a heart attack. It occurs when there is myocardial necrosis following atherosclerotic plaque rupture, which occludes one or more of the coronary arteries. MI is part of the acute coronary syndromes.
The acute coronary syndromes comprise:
- ST elevation MI (STEMI).
- Non-ST elevation MI (NSTEMI).
- Unstable angina.

Causes
- Atherosclerosis.

Symptoms
- Nausea, sweating, palpitations.
- Crushing chest pain for more than 20 minutes.
- N.B. Can be silent in diabetics.

Signs
Remember these as **RIP**:
- **R**aised jugular venous pressure (JVP).
- **I**ncreased pulse, blood pressure changes.
- **P**allor, anxiety.

Pathophysiology
See page 9 for the pathophysiology of atherosclerosis.

Treatment

- Conservative: lifestyle measures such as smoking cessation and increased exercise.
- Medical – **MONA B** for immediate management:
  - **Morphine.**
  - **Oxygen** (if hypoxic).
  - **Nitrates** (glyceryl trinitrate [GTN]).
  - **Anticoagulants**, e.g. aspirin and an antiemetic.
  - **Beta-blockers** if no contraindication.

On discharge all patients should be prescribed: aspirin, an angiotensin converting enzyme (ACE) inhibitor, a beta-blocker (if no contraindication; calcium channel blockers are good alternatives) and a statin.

- Surgical: reperfusion with PCI if STEMI. PCI may also be used in NSTEMI but if NSTEMI patients are not having immediate PCI, fondaparinux (a factor Xa inhibitor) or a low molecular weight heparin (LMWH) may be given subcutaneously.

Complications

Remember this as **C PEAR DROP**:

- **C**ardiogenic shock, **C**ardiac arrhythmia.

N.B. Atrial fibrillation (AF) increases a patient's risk of stroke. AF presents with an irregularly irregular pulse and an ECG with absent P waves, irregular RR intervals, an undulating baseline and narrow QRS complexes. Start anticoagulation therapy.

- **P**ericarditis.
- **E**mboli.
- **A**neurysm formation.
- **R**upture of ventricle.
- **D**ressler's syndrome: an autoimmune pericarditis that develops 2–10 weeks post MI. This is a triad of: 1) fever; 2) pleuritic pain; 3) pericardial effusion.
- **R**upture of free wall.
- **O**
- **P**apillary muscle rupture.

Map 1.3 Myocardial Infarction (MI)

The Cardiovascular System

Map 1.4 Angina Pectoris

What is angina pectoris?

Angina pectoris may be defined as substernal discomfort that is precipitated by exercise but relieved by rest or GTN spray.

Causes
- Atherosclerosis.
- Rarely anaemia and tachyarrhythmia.

Precipitants
- Exercise.
- Cold weather.
- Heavy meals.

Types of angina

- Stable angina: precipitated by exercise but relieved by rest.
  ST DEPRESSION
- Unstable angina: pain at rest, worsening symptoms.
  ST DEPRESSION
- Decubitus angina: triggered by lying flat.
  ST DEPRESSION
- Prinzmetal angina: due to coronary artery spasm.
  ST ELEVATION

Investigations: ECG

- **ECG** for signs of ST depression or ST elevation. Exercise ECG is no longer recommended by NICE guidelines.
- **CT** scan, **C**oronary **C**alcium Score (this is measured on CT) and Coronary angiography.
- **G**o for thallium scan.

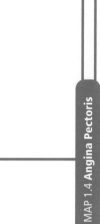

MAP 1.4 Angina Pectoris

Pathophysiology of atherosclerosis

Atherosclerosis is a slowly progressive disease and is the underlying cause of ischaemic heart disease when it occurs in the coronary arteries.

There are 3 stages of atheroma formation:

1 Fatty streak formation

Lipids are deposited in the intimal layer of the artery. This, coupled with vascular injury, causes inflammation, increased permeability and white blood cell recruitment. Macrophages phagocytose the lipid and become foam cells. These form the fatty streak.

2 Fibrolipid plaque formation

Lipid within the intimal layer stimulates the formation of fibrocollagenous tissue. This eventually causes thinning of the muscular media.

3 Complicated atheroma

This occurs when the plaque is extensive and prone to rupture. The plaque may be calcified due to lipid acquisition of calcium. Rupture activates clot formation and thrombosis. If the coronary artery is partially occluded the result is myocardial ischaemia and therefore angina. If the coronary artery is completely occluded then the result is myocardial necrosis and MI.

Complications

- MI.
- Stroke.

Treatment

- Conservative: modify risk factors, e.g. control cholesterol, control diabetes, smoking cessation advice, weight loss, increase exercise and control hypertension.
- Medical:
  - Nitrates: glyceryl trinitrate (GTN) spray. Side-effects include headache and hypotension.
  - **A – Aspirin.**
  - **B – Beta-blockers** but contraindicated in asthma and chronic obstructive pulmonary disease (COPD).
  - **C – Ca²⁺ antagonists** especially if beta-blockers are contraindicated.
  - K⁺ channel activator, e.g. nicorandil.
- Surgery: percutaneous transluminal coronary angioplasty or coronary artery bypass graft (CABG).

Map 1.4 Angina Pectoris

Map 1.5 Infective Endocarditis

What is infective endocarditis?

It is an infection of the endocardium usually involving the heart valves, with 'vegetation' of the infectious agent.

The mitral valve is more commonly affected but the tricuspid valve is implicated in IV drug users.

Risk factors

- IV drug abuse.
- Cardiac lesions.
- Rheumatic heart disease.
- Dental treatment: requires antibiotic prophylaxis.

Pathophysiology

Infective endocarditis is a rare infection that usually affects patients who already have a structural valve abnormality. The reason why heart valves are targeted is because the valves of the heart have limited blood supply and consequently white blood cells cannot reach the valves through the blood. Circulating bacteria adhere to the valve causing vegetations.

Classification of infective endocarditis

Duke Criteria: 2 major criteria *or* 1 major and 3 minor criteria *or* 5 minor criteria.

- Major criteria:
  - 2 separate positive blood cultures.
  - Endocardial involvement.
- Minor criteria: **FIVE**
  - Fever >38°C.
  - **IV** drug user or predisposing heart condition, and
  - Immunological phenomena, e.g. Osler's nodes or Roth's spots.
  - **Vascular phenomena, e.g. mycotic aneurysm or Janeway lesions.**
  - **Echocardiograph findings.**

Investigations

- Blood cultures: take 3 separate cultures from 3 peripheral sites.
- Bloods for anaemia.
- Urinalysis; microscopic haematuria.
- CXR.
- Transoesophageal/ transthoracic ECHO for vegetations.

Causative agents

- *Streptococcus viridans.*
- *Staphylococcus aureus.*
- *Staphylococcus epidermidis.*
- Diphtheroids.
- Microaerophilic streptococci.
- HACEK group: *Haemophilus, Actinobacillus, Cardiobacterium, Eikenella and Kingella.*

MAP 1.5
Infective Endocarditis

Treatment

Depends on the causative agent. Check hospital antibiotic guidelines.

- Conservative: maintain good oral hygiene.
- Medical: empirical therapy is **benzylpenicillin** and **gentamicin**.
  - Streptococci: **benzylpenicillin** and **amoxicillin**.
  - Staphylococci: **flucloxacillin** and **gentamicin**.
  - *Aspergillus*: **miconazole**.
- Surgical: valve repair or valve replacement.

Complications

- Heart failure.
- Arrhythmias.
- Abscess formation in the cardiac muscle.
- Emboli formation: may cause stroke, vision loss or spread the infection to other regions of the body.

Signs and symptoms

Remember this as **FROM JANE:**

- **F**ever.
- **R**oth's spots (seen on fundoscopy).
- **O**sler's nodes (painful nodules seen on the fingers and toes).
- new **M**urmur.

- **J**aneway lesions (painless papules seen on the palms and plantars).
- **A**naemia.
- **N**ails: splinter haemorrhages.
- **E**mboli.

FIGURE 1.1 **Heart Valves**

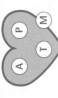

Remember the heart valves as:
All Prostitutes Take Money
(Aortic, Pulmonary, Tricuspid, Mitral).

The Cardiovascular System

Map 1.5 Infective Endocarditis

Table 1.1 Aortic Valve Disease

TABLE 1.1 Aortic Valve Disease

Valve lesion	Causes	Symptoms	Signs	Murmur	Investigations	Treatment	Complications
Aortic stenosis	Atherosclerotic-like calcific degeneration Congenital bicuspid valve Rheumatic heart disease	Syncope Dyspnoea Angina	Narrow pulse pressure Slow rising pulse	Crescendo-decrescendo ejection systolic murmur, which radiates to the carotids	ECG: left ventricular hypertrophy; AV block CXR: poststenotic dilation of the ascending aorta; may see calcification of valve on lateral view ECHO: confirms diagnosis; allows severity and valve area to be assessed	Conservative: manage cardiovascular risk factors, e.g. smoking cessation Medical: manage cardiovascular risk factors, e.g. control blood pressure Surgical: valve replacement is the treatment of choice	Sudden death Arrhythmia Heart failure Infective endocarditis
Aortic regurgitation	**Acute** Cusp rupture Connective tissue disorders,	Dyspnoea Angina Heart failure	Waterhammer pulse Wide pulse pressure	Decrescendo early diastolic murmur	ECG: left ventricular hypertrophy	Conservative: manage cardiovascular risk factors, e.g. smoking cessation	Heart failure Arrhythmia Infective endocarditis

e.g. Marfan's syndrome Aortic dissection Perforation secondary to infection **Chronic** Rheumatoid arthritis Ankylosing spondylitis Syphilis	Traube's sign: a 'pistol shot' heard over the femoral artery De Musset's sign: head nodding in time with heart beat Quincke's sign: pulse felt in the nail Signs of systemic disease	CXR: may see cardiomegaly and pulmonary oedema if patient has heart failure ECHO: confirms diagnosis; allows severity and aortic root to be assessed	Medical: manage heart failure by following NICE guidelines Surgical: valve replacement is the treatment of choice

Table 1.1 Aortic Valve Disease

TABLE 1.2 **Mitral Valve Disease**

Valve lesion	Causes	Symptoms	Signs	Murmur	Investigations	Treatment	Complications
Mitral stenosis	Rheumatic heart disease Calcification of valve Rheumatoid arthritis Ankylosing spondylitis Systemic lupus erythematosus (SLE) Malignant carcinoid	Dyspnoea Palpitations if in atrial fibrillation (AF) Heart failure Haemoptysis	Malar flush Tapping apex beat Hoarse voice (Ortner's syndrome) Irregularly irregular pulse if in AF	Low pitch mid-diastolic murmur with opening snap	ECG: atrial fibrillation; bifid P waves CXR: pulmonary oedema and enlarged left atrium may be seen ECHO: confirms diagnosis; allows severity and valve area to be assessed	Conservative: manage cardiovascular risk factors, e.g. smoking cessation Medical: manage AF and heart failure by following NICE guidelines Surgical: valve replacement is the treatment of choice	AF Heart failure Infective endocarditis
Mitral regurgitation	Rheumatic heart disease Papillary muscle rupture Infective endocarditis Prolapse	Dyspnoea Palpitations if in AF Heart failure Symptoms of infective endocarditis	Irregularly irregular pulse if in AF Displaced apex beat	A harsh pansystolic murmur radiating to the axilla	ECG: atrial fibrillation; bifid P waves CXR: may see cardiomegaly and pulmonary oedema if patient has heart failure	Conservative: manage cardiovascular risk factors, e.g. smoking cessation	AF Heart failure Infective endocarditis Pulmonary hypertension

Table 1.2 Mitral Valve Disease

| | | | | ECHO: confirms diagnosis; allows severity to be assessed | Medical: manage heart failure and AF by following NICE guidelines

Surgical: valve repair is preferred since replacement may interfere with the function of the papillary muscles |
|---|---|---|---|---|---|

Table 1.2 Mitral Valve Disease

What is hypertension?

This is a clinic blood pressure that is >140/90 mmHg.

Pathophysiology

There is much uncertainty as to the cause of hypertension but it is likely multifactorial. ~95% of cases have no known cause and, in these cases, patients are said to have 'essential hypertension'.

More rarely, patients will have secondary hypertension. This should be considered in young patients with an acute onset of hypertension, any history that is suggestive of a renal or endocrine cause and when the patient fails to respond to medical therapy. Examples include renovascular disease, Conn's syndrome, Cushing's disease and phaeochromocytoma.

Blood pressure is controlled by several mechanisms, e.g. the autonomic nervous system, the capillary fluid shift mechanism, the renin angiotensin aldosterone system and adrenaline. A problem with one of these mechanisms may result in high blood pressure.

Lifestyle factors such as smoking, alcohol intake, obesity and stress also play a role in increasing blood pressure.

Investigations

- Clinic blood pressure readings (with ambulatory blood pressure monitoring to confirm). Stages of hypertension are listed below:

Blood pressure (mmHg)	Systolic	Diastolic
Normal	<120	<80
Pre-hypertension	120–139	80–89
Stage 1	140–159	90–99
Stage 2	160–179	100–109
Severe hypertension	≥180	≥110

- Bloods: FBC, LFTs, U&Es, creatinine, serum urea, eGFR, lipid levels and glucose.
- ECG: left ventricular hypertrophy.
- Urine dipstick: haematuria and proteinuria.

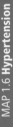

MAP 1.6 **Hypertension**

Causes

- Unknown: 'essential hypertension'.
- Secondary causes: renal and endocrine disease.
- Contributory lifestyle factors such as increased stress, smoking and obesity.

Complications

- MI.
- Heart failure.
- Renal impairment.
- Stroke.
- Hypertensive retinopathy.

Treatment

- Conservative: lifestyle advice including smoking cessation, encouraging weight loss, decreased alcohol consumption and a salt restricted diet.
- Medical: this is split into 4 steps according to NICE guidelines:

	<55 years old		>55 years old/black patients
Step 1	A	C	or	C	D
Step 2	A + C	or	C + D
Step 3	A + C + D		
Step 4	Refer for add-on therapy		

Key:
A: angiotensin converting enzyme (ACE) inhibitor or angiotensin receptor blocker (ARB) if ACE inhibitor is not tolerated by patient;
C: calcium channel blocker;
D: thiazide-type diuretic;
add-on therapy: spironolactone (side-effect: hyperkalaemia), alpha-blocker or beta-blocker.

- Surgical: surgical excision (if related to cause).

FIGURE 1.2 The Renin Angiotensin System

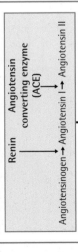

Renin → Angiotensin converting enzyme (ACE) →

Angiotensinogen → Angiotensin I → Angiotensin II

Angiotensin II stimulates:
- Aldosterone secretion from the zona glomerulosa of the adrenal cortex.
- Vasoconstriction.
- Antidiuretic hormone (ADH) release from the posterior pituitary gland.
- The sympathetic system.

Map 1.7 Atrial Fibrillation (AF)

What is AF?

This is the most common tachyarrhythmia, characterised by an irregularly irregular pulse, rapid heart rate and ECG changes.

Signs and symptoms

- None.
- Palpitations.
- Dyspnoea.
- Syncope.
- Exercise intolerance.
- Fatigue.
- Heart failure.
- Irregularly irregular pulse.

Pathophysiology

Atrial ectopic beats, thought to originate in the pulmonary veins, lead to dysfunction of the cardiac electrical signalling pathway. As a result the atria no longer contract in a coordinated manner. Instead they fibrillate and contract irregularly. Due to the irregular contractions, the atria fail to empty adequately. This may result in stagnant blood accumulating within the atrial appendage, increasing the risk of clot formation and therefore embolic stroke.

Investigations

- ECG: absent P waves, irregular RR intervals, an undulating baseline and narrow QRS complexes.
- Holter monitoring: ambulatory ECG device.
- ECHO.
- TFTs.
- CXR.

MAP 1.7 Atrial Fibrillation (AF)

Treatment

- Conservative: patient education and management of cardiovascular risk factors, e.g. smoking cessation and decreasing alcohol intake.
- Medical: treat underlying cause and:
  ○ Restore rate: beta-blocker, calcium antagonist, digoxin, amiodarone.
  ○ Restore rhythm: beta-blocker, cardioversion, amiodarone.
  ○ Anticoagulant, e.g. warfarin, apixaban, dabigatran and rivaroxaban (see Appendix 2).

Complications

- Stroke.
- Heart failure.
- Sudden death.

Causes

- Idiopathic.
- Ischaemic heart disease.
- Heart failure.
- Valve disease: mitral stenosis and mitral regurgitation.
- Hypertension.
- Hyperthyroidism.
- Alcohol induced.
- Familial.

The Respiratory System

What is pneumonia?

Pneumonia is inflammation of the lung parenchyma caused by a lower respiratory tract infection. It often occurs after a viral infection in the upper respiratory tract. It is uncertain how the bacteria reach the lower respiratory tract after attaching to disaccharide receptors on pharyngeal epithelial cells.

Pathophysiology

Debatable methods of invasion include:

- The inhibition of IgA.
- Pneumolysins, which inhibit ciliary beating.
- Damage of the epithelial cells by prior infection.
- Hijacking the platelet aggregating factor receptor pathway to reach the alveoli.

Symptoms

- Fever.
- Cough with purulent sputum.
- Dyspnoea.
- Pleuritic pain.

Signs

- Percussion: dull.
- Auscultation: crackles, bronchial breathing.
- Respiratory failure: cyanosis, tachypnoea.
- Septicaemia: rigors.

Causative organisms

	Community acquired pneumonia	Hospital acquired pneumonia	HIV patients or immunocompromised patients
Children	Streptococcus pneumoniae	Gram-negative bacteria	Pneumocystis jirovecii
Pneumococcus	Haemophilus influenzae	Staphylococcus aureus	Cytomegalovirus
Mycoplasma	Moraxella catarrhalis	Streptococcus pneumoniae	Adenovirus
	Chlamydia pneumoniae (A)	Anaerobes	Herpes simplex virus
	Mycoplasma pneumoniae (A)	Fungi	Mycobacterium tuberculosis
	Legionella pneumophila (A)	Legionella pneumophila	Bacterial infection, e.g. Staphylococcus aureus
	Viruses		

A = Atypical

MAP 2.1 **Pneumonia**

Treatment

Remember this as **BAPP**:

- **B**reathing: maintain oxygen saturation levels.
- **A**ntibiotics: treat the underlying cause (check hospital guidelines).
- **P**ain: give analgesics.
- **P**neumococcal vaccines for those at risk, e.g. diabetics, the immunosuppressed and those over 65 years old.

Complications

- Respiratory failure: by causing acute respiratory distress syndrome (ARDS).
- Septic shock: the causative agent enters the patient's bloodstream, releasing cytokines.
- Pleural effusion.
- Empyema.
- Lung abscess.
- Hypotension: sepsis or dehydration is usually the underlying cause.

Investigations

- CXR: look for infiltrates.
- Identify the causative organism by assessing a sputum sample.
- Monitor oxygen saturation.
- Bloods: look for raised WCC and raised inflammatory markers.
- Urinary antigen test: for pneumococcal or *Legionella* antigen.
- Arterial blood gas (ABG).

Assess **severity** using **CURB-65**
- **C**onfusion.
- **U**rea >7 mmol/L.
- **R**espiratory rate >30/min.
- **B**P <90/<60 mmHg.
- >**65** years old.

Each section of the CURB-65 is worth 1 point:
- 1 = Outpatient care.
- 2 = Admission.
- >3 = Requires ICU admission.

Map 2.2 Bronchiectasis

What is bronchiectasis?

Bronchiectasis is permanent dilation of the airways caused by chronic inflammation and inability to clear secretions.

Pathophysiology

This is dependent on the cause. Initially, there is infection of the smaller distal airways that results in inflammation and the release of inflammatory mediators. This impairs ciliary action, allows for bacterial proliferation and tissue damage and causes bronchial dilation.

Causes

- Congenital:
  ○ Cystic fibrosis.
  ○ Young's syndrome: associated with azoospermia.
  ○ Kartagener's syndrome: causes cilia to become immobile, thus removing the defence mechanism of the respiratory tract; also associated with situs inversus.
- Acquired:
  ○ Tumours.
  ○ Rheumatoid arthritis.
  ○ Inflammatory bowel disease.

MAP 2.2 Bronchiectasis

Complications

- Massive haemoptysis: this is a medical emergency.

Causative organisms

- *Streptococcus pneumoniae.*
- *Haemophilus influenzae.*
- *Staphylococcus aureus.*
- *Pseudomonas aeruginosa:* common in patients with cystic fibrosis.

Investigations

- Bloods: FBC, WCC, U&Es, LFTs, TFTs, CRP, ESR.
- CXR: shows tram track opacities of bronchi and bronchioles.
- Sputum culture and sensitivity.
- *Aspergillus* screen if cause suspected.

Symptoms

- Purulent sputum.
- Persistent cough.
- Fever.

Signs

- Clubbing.
- Crepitations.
- Coarse inspiratory crackles.

Treatment

Remember this as **ABCDS**:

- **A**ntibiotics.
- **B**ronchodilators.
- **C**orticosteroids.
- postural **D**rainage.
- **S**urgery (if indicated).

CYSTIC FIBROSIS

What is cystic fibrosis?

This is an autosomal recessive condition that occurs in approximately 1 in 2500 births.

Causes

- Mutation of the cystic fibrosis transmembrane conductance regulator gene (*CFTR*), located on chromosome 7.

Investigations

- Diagnosed by sweat test.
- In the neonatal period diagnosed by Guthrie's test, which detects raised serum immunoreactive trypsinogen.

Associations

- Lung disease, pancreatic insufficiency, diabetes and infertility in males.

Map 2.2 Bronchiectasis

What is asthma?

Asthma is a **chronic, inflammatory** disease that is characterised by **reversible** airway obstruction.

Signs and symptoms

- Wheezing.
- Shortness of breath.
- Coughing.

Remember to ask if the patient has a history of atopy, e.g. hay fever and eczema.

Triggering factors include:

- Dust/pets/vapours.
- Emotion.
- Drugs, e.g. beta-blockers.

Investigations

- Peak expiratory flow rate: note diurnal variation.
- Sputum sample.
- ABG: in emergency.
- Spirometry: for obstructive defects.
- Bloods: increased IgE, FBC.
- CXR: pneumothorax, consolidation.

Pathophysiology

- Copious mucus secretion.
- Inflammation.
- Contraction of bronchial muscle.

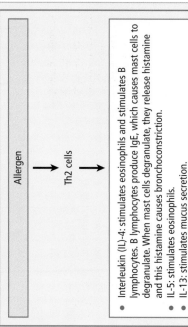

Allergen → Th2 cells →

- Interleukin (IL)-4: stimulates eosinophils and stimulates B lymphocytes. B lymphocytes produce IgE, which causes mast cells to degranulate. When mast cells degranulate, they release histamine and this histamine causes bronchoconstriction.
- IL-5: stimulates eosinophils.
- IL-13: stimulates mucus secretion.

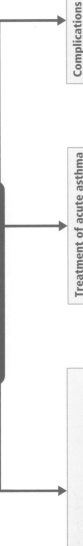

MAP 2.3 Asthma

Complications
- Death.
- Disturbed sleep.
- Persistent cough.
- Side-effects of steroids:
  - Weight gain.
  - Thinning of the skin.
  - Striae formation.
  - Cataracts.
  - Cushing's syndrome.

Treatment of acute asthma
Remember as **O SHIT**:
- **O**xygen.

- **S**albutamol.
- **H**ydrocortisone.
- **I**pratropium.
- **T**heophylline.

Treatment
- Conservative: patient education; advice on inhaler technique and avoidance of triggering factors; annual asthma review and influenza vaccine required.
- Medical: refer to British Thoracic Society Guidelines:
  - Step 1: salbutamol (a short-acting beta-2 receptor agonist).
  - Step 2: step 1 + beclometasone (inhaled steroid).
  - Step 3: steps 1, 2 + salmeterol (a long-acting beta-2 receptor agonist) + increased total dose of inhaled steroid.
  - Step 4: steps 1–3 + increased dose of inhaled steroid + consider adding additional therapy, e.g.:
    - Theophylline (a xanthine derived bronchodilator that inhibits phosphodiesterase).
    - Montelukast (a leukotriene receptor antagonist).
  - Step 5: oral prednisolone (steroid) + high-dose inhaled steroid; refer to specialist.

Map 2.4 Chronic Obstructive Pulmonary Disease (COPD)

Pathophysiology

- Chronic bronchitis: chronic infection results in the chronic infiltration of the respiratory submucosa by inflammatory cells. This results in mucous gland hyperplasia and smooth muscle hypertrophy, causing bronchial lumen narrowing. 'Blue bloaters' are patients where this pathology dominates.

- Emphysema: alveolar walls are destroyed resulting in bullae formation and the fusion of adjacent alveoli. This ultimately results in a decreased surface area for gas exchange and decreased elastic recoil with subsequent air trapping. 'Pink puffers' are patients where this pathology dominates.

Causes

Remember this as **GASES**:

- **G**enetics: alpha-1 antitrypsin deficiency results in the loss of protection against proteases.
- **A**ir pollution.
- **S**moking.
- **E**xposure through occupation, e.g. coal mining.
- **S**econdhand smoke exposure.

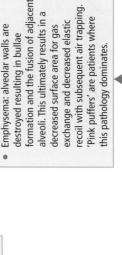

MAP 2.4 **Chronic Obstructive Pulmonary Disease (COPD)**

What is COPD?

This is a chronic obstructive airway disease that is characterised by its irreversibility. It is closely linked to smoking.
It is made up of:

- Chronic bronchitis: cough with sputum production for at least 3 months in 2 consecutive years.
- Emphysema: this encompasses permanently dilated airways distal to the terminal bronchioles with alveolar destruction and bullae formation. It is defined histologically and is associated with alpha-1 antitrypsin deficiency and increased elastase activity.

Investigations

- Diagnosis is confirmed by spirometry, which has a FEV_1 value <80% predicted and FEV_1/FVC <0.7.
- CXR shows lung hyperinflation, emphysematous change and diaphragmatic flattening.
- Bloods: FBC, U&Es, WCC, ESR, CRP, alpha-1 antitrypsin levels.
- ECG: for cor pulmonale.
- Sputum culture.

The **GOLD scale** assesses severity of COPD:

Stage I: mild COPD.
Stage II: moderate COPD.
Stage III: severe COPD.
Stage IV: very severe COPD.

Complications

Remember this as **CLIPPeR**:

- **C**or pulmonale: right-sided heart failure due to chronic pulmonary hypertension.
- **L**ung cancer.
- **I**nfections: usually treat with macrolide antibiotics.
- **P**neumothorax.
- **P**olycythaemia.
- **e**
- **R**espiratory failure.

Treatment

Remember this as **ABCS, oxygen therapy and pulmonary rehabilitation**:

- **A**nticholinergics, e.g. ipratropium.
- **B**ronchodilators, e.g. salmeterol.
- **C**orticosteroids.
- **S**moking cessation is imperative.
- **Oxygen therapy**: long-term oxygen therapy (LTOT) or noninvasive ventilation (NIV).

Map 2.4 Chronic Obstructive Pulmonary Disease (COPD)

Table 2.1 Type 1 vs. Type 2 Respiratory Failure

TABLE 2.1 Type 1 vs. Type 2 Respiratory Failure

	Type 1: hypoventilation with V/Q mismatch 'Pink puffer' – thin and hyperinflated	Type 2: hypoventilation with or without V/Q mismatch 'Blue bloater' – strong build and wheezy
Cause	Pneumonia Pulmonary embolism Pulmonary oedema Fibrosing alveolitis	Chronic obstructive pulmonary disease (COPD) and asthma Cerebrovascular disease Opiate overdose Myasthenia gravis Motor neuron disease
Symptoms	Remember this as **ABCD**: **A**gitation **B**reathlessness **C**onfusion **D**rowsiness and fatigue	Remember this as **ABCD**: **A**gitation **B**reathlessness **C**onfusion **D**rowsiness and fatigue
Signs	Central cyanosis	Remember this as **ABC**: **A** flapping tremor **B**ounding pulse **C**yanosis
PaO_2	$\downarrow$ (<8.0 kPa)	$\downarrow$ (<8.0 kPa)
$PaCO_2$	Normal (~6.7 kPa)	$\uparrow$ (>6.7 kPa)
Treatment	Oxygen replacement therapy Treatment of underlying cause	Noninvasive ventilation Treatment of underlying cause
Complications	Nosocomial infections, e.g. pneumonia Heart failure Arrhythmia Pericarditis	Nosocomial infections, e.g. pneumonia Heart failure Arrhythmia Pericarditis

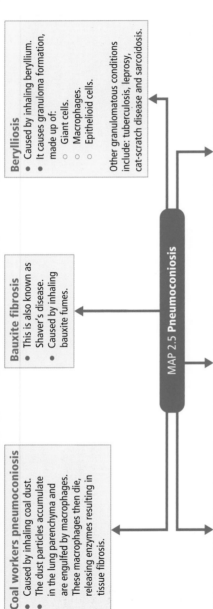

MAP 2.5 Pneumoconiosis

Coal workers pneumoconiosis
- Caused by inhaling coal dust.
- The dust particles accumulate in the lung parenchyma and are engulfed by macrophages. These macrophages then die, releasing enzymes resulting in tissue fibrosis.

Bauxite fibrosis
- This is also known as Shaver's disease.
- Caused by inhaling bauxite fumes.

Berylliosis
- Caused by inhaling beryllium.
- It causes granuloma formation, made up of:
  ○ Giant cells.
  ○ Macrophages.
  ○ Epithelioid cells.

Other granulomatous conditions include: tuberculosis, leprosy, cat-scratch disease and sarcoidosis.

Asbestosis
- Caused by inhaling asbestos fibres. The fusiform rods are found inside macrophages.
- Associated with malignant mesothelioma.
- Pleural plaques are apparent on CXR.
- White asbestos has the lowest fibrogenicity, whereas blue asbestos has the highest.

Siderosis
- Caused by inhaling iron particles.
- Benign with no apparent respiratory symptoms or altered lung function.

Silicosis
- This is also known as Potter's rot.
- Caused by inhaling silica particles, which cannot be removed by respiratory defences.
- Macrophages engulf the silica particles releasing tumour necrosis factor (TNF) and cytokines that induce fibroblasts, resulting in fibrosis and collagen deposition.
- Associated with increased tuberculosis (TB) infection.
- Eggshell calcification of hilar lymph nodes is apparent on CXR, along with nodular lesions in the upper lobes.

Map 2.5 Pneumoconiosis

Map 2.6 Lung Cancer

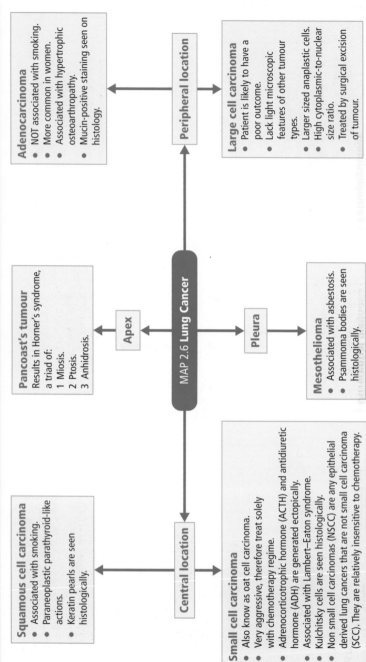

MAP 2.6 Lung Cancer

Peripheral location

Adenocarcinoma
- NOT associated with smoking.
- More common in women.
- Associated with hypertrophic osteoarthropathy.
- Mucin-positive staining seen on histology.

Large cell carcinoma
- Patient is likely to have a poor outcome.
- Lack light microscopic features of other tumour types.
- Larger sized anaplastic cells.
- High cytoplasmic-to-nuclear size ratio.
- Treated by surgical excision of tumour.

Apex

Pancoast's tumour
Results in Horner's syndrome, a triad of:
1 Miosis.
2 Ptosis.
3 Anhidrosis.

Pleura

Mesothelioma
- Associated with asbestosis.
- Psammoma bodies are seen histologically.

Central location

Squamous cell carcinoma
- Associated with smoking.
- Paraneoplastic parathyroid-like actions.
- Keratin pearls are seen histologically.

Small cell carcinoma
- Also know as oat cell carcinoma.
- Very aggressive, therefore treat solely with chemotherapy regime.
- Adrenocorticotrophic hormone (ACTH) and antidiuretic hormone (ADH) are generated ectopically.
- Associated with Lambert–Eaton syndrome.
- Kulchitsky cells are seen histologically.
- Non small cell carcinomas (NSCC) are any epithelial derived lung cancers that are not small cell carcinoma (SCC). They are relatively insensitive to chemotherapy.

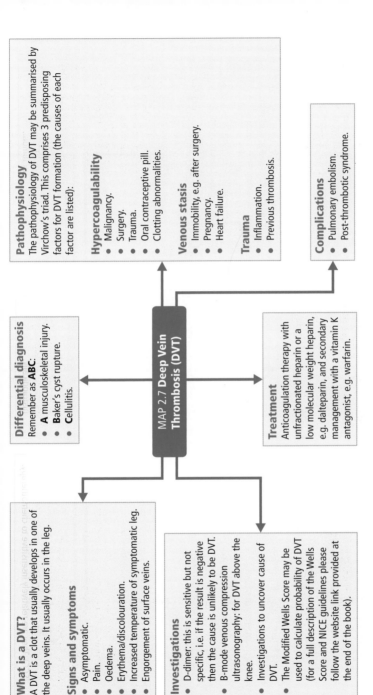

Pathophysiology

The pathophysiology of DVT may be summarised by Virchow's triad. This comprises 3 predisposing factors for DVT formation (the causes of each factor are listed):

Hypercoagulability
- Malignancy.
- Surgery.
- Trauma.
- Oral contraceptive pill.
- Clotting abnormalities.

Venous stasis
- Immobility, e.g. after surgery.
- Pregnancy.
- Heart failure.

Trauma
- Inflammation.
- Previous thrombosis.

Complications
- Pulmonary embolism.
- Post-thrombotic syndrome.

Differential diagnosis
Remember as **ABC**:
- **A** musculoskeletal injury.
- **B**aker's cyst rupture.
- **C**ellulitis.

Treatment
Anticoagulation therapy with unfractionated heparin or a low molecular weight heparin, e.g. dalteparin, and secondary management with a vitamin K antagonist, e.g. warfarin.

MAP 2.7 Deep Vein Thrombosis (DVT)

What is a DVT?
A DVT is a clot that usually develops in one of the deep veins. It usually occurs in the leg.

Signs and symptoms
- Asymptomatic.
- Pain.
- Oedema.
- Erythema/discolouration.
- Increased temperature of symptomatic leg.
- Engorgement of surface veins.

Investigations
- D-dimer: this is sensitive but not specific, i.e. if the result is negative then the cause is unlikely to be DVT.
- B-mode venous compression ultrasonography: for DVT above the knee.
- Investigations to uncover cause of DVT.
- The Modified Wells Score may be used to calculate probability of DVT (for a full description of the Wells Score and NICE guidelines please follow the website link provided at the end of the book).

Map 2.7 Deep Vein Thrombosis (DVT)

Map 2.8 Pulmonary Embolism (PE)

Pathophysiology

The extent of thrombus may be classified into small-medium, multiple and massive PE. Symptom correlation depends on where the pulmonary circulation is occluded.

There are 3 pathways involved in the pathophysiology of PE:
1 Platelet factor release: serotonin and thromboxane A_2 cause vasoconstriction.
2 Decreased alveolar perfusion: lung is underperfused and this leads to diminished gas exchange.
3 Decreased surfactant: this leads to ventilation/perfusion mismatch, hypoxaemia and dyspnoea.

Causes

- DVT.
- Air embolus.
- Fat embolus.
- Amniotic fluid embolus.
- Foreign material introduced via IV drug use.

What is a PE?

This is occlusion of the pulmonary vasculature by a clot. Often it occurs from a deep vein thrombosis (DVT) that has become dislodged and forms an embolus that lodges in the pulmonary arterial vasculature, blocking the vessels.

Signs and symptoms

- Breathlessness: this may be of sudden onset or progressive.
- Tachypnoea.
- Pleuritic chest pain.
- Cyanosis.
- Haemoptysis.

MAP 2.8 **Pulmonary Embolism (PE)**

Investigations

- D-dimer: sensitive but not specific; negative result used to rule out PE.
- Thrombophilia screening: in patients <50 years with recurrent PE.
- CXR: usually normal.
- ECG: sinus tachycardia, S1Q3T3 pattern is classical but rare; excludes MI.
- ABG: hypoxaemia.
- CT, pulmonary angiography.
- V/Q scan.
- The Wells Score may be used to calculate risk of PE.

Treatment

- Acute:
  - Oxygen.
  - IV fluids.
  - Thrombolysis therapy if indicated, e.g. alteplase if massive PE or haemodynamically unstable.
  - Low molecular weight heparin.
- Long-term management:
  - Anticoagulation.
  - Inferior vena cava filter.

Complications

- Sudden death.
- Arrhythmia.
- Pulmonary infarction.
- Pleural effusion.
- Paradoxical embolism.
- Pulmonary hypertension.

Map 2.9 Pneumothorax

MAP 2.9 Pneumothorax

What is a pneumothorax?
A pneumothorax is air within the pleural space.

Signs and symptoms
- Ipsilateral chest pain.
- Shoulder tip pain.
- Dyspnoea.
- Tachypnoea.
- Hypoxia.
- Cyanosis.
- Auscultation: decreased on affected side.
- Percussion: hyper-resonant or normal.

Investigations
- CXR: pleural line; may show tracheal deviation away from lesion.
- CT scan.
- ABG: hypoxia.

Causes
- Ruptured pleural bleb.
- Chronic obstructive pulmonary disease (COPD).
- Tuberculosis.
- Sarcoidosis.
- Idiopathic pulmonary fibrosis.
- Rheumatoid arthritis.
- Ankylosing spondylitis.
- Lung cancer.
- Trauma, e.g. stab wound.

Pathophysiology
The pathophysiology of pneumothorax is directly linked to cause, outlined below.
- Primary spontaneous pneumothorax:
  - Idiopathic/rupture of pleural bleb.
  - Usually found in young, tall, slim men.
- Secondary spontaneous pneumothorax:
  - In patients with prior lung disease, e.g. COPD, sarcoidosis or idiopathic pulmonary fibrosis.
- Tension pneumothorax:
  - Due to blunt, traumatic injuries, e.g. a stab wound.
  - Air cannot be removed on expiration due to one-way valve mechanism. This leads to mediastinal shift and lung collapse.

Treatment
- If pneumothorax on CXR <2 cm then no treatment is required; advise patients not to travel by air or to dive.
- If >2 cm then aspirate air +/– intercostal drain.
- Tension pneumothorax requires immediate decompression with a large bore needle inserted into the 2nd intercostal space mid-clavicular line.

Complications
- Risk of future pneumothorax.
- Respiratory failure.
- Cardiac arrest.

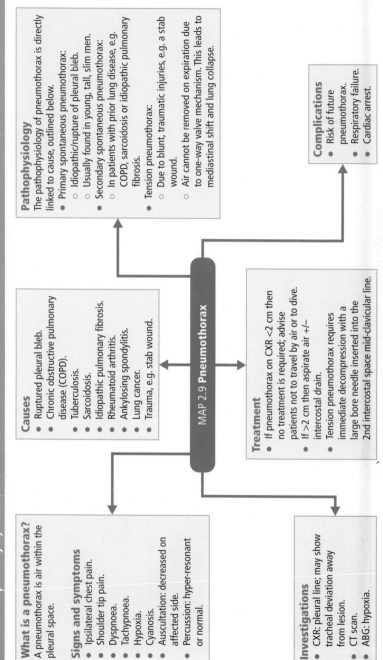

Map 3.1 Causes of Regional Abdominal Pain

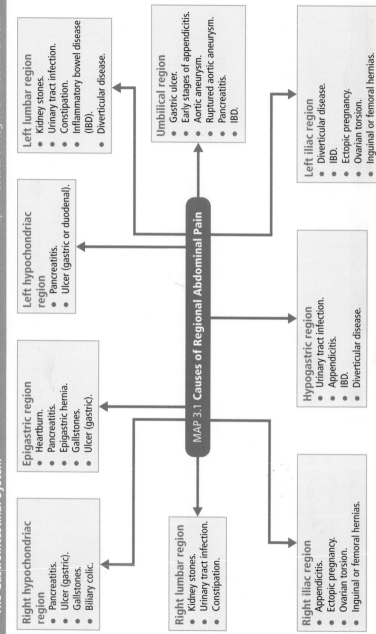

MAP 3.1 Causes of Regional Abdominal Pain

Right hypochondriac region
- Pancreatitis.
- Ulcer (gastric).
- Gallstones.
- Biliary colic.

Epigastric region
- Heartburn.
- Pancreatitis.
- Epigastric hernia.
- Gallstones.
- Ulcer (gastric).

Left hypochondriac region
- Pancreatitis.
- Ulcer (gastric or duodenal).

Left lumbar region
- Kidney stones.
- Urinary tract infection.
- Constipation.
- Inflammatory bowel disease (IBD).
- Diverticular disease.

Umbilical region
- Gastric ulcer.
- Early stages of appendicitis.
- Aortic aneurysm.
- Ruptured aortic aneurysm.
- Pancreatitis.
- IBD.

Right lumbar region
- Kidney stones.
- Urinary tract infection.
- Constipation.

Hypogastric region
- Urinary tract infection.
- Appendicitis.
- IBD.
- Diverticular disease.

Left iliac region
- Diverticular disease.
- IBD.
- Ectopic pregnancy.
- Ovarian torsion.
- Inguinal or femoral hernias.

Right iliac region
- Appendicitis.
- Ectopic pregnancy.
- Ovarian torsion.
- Inguinal or femoral hernias.

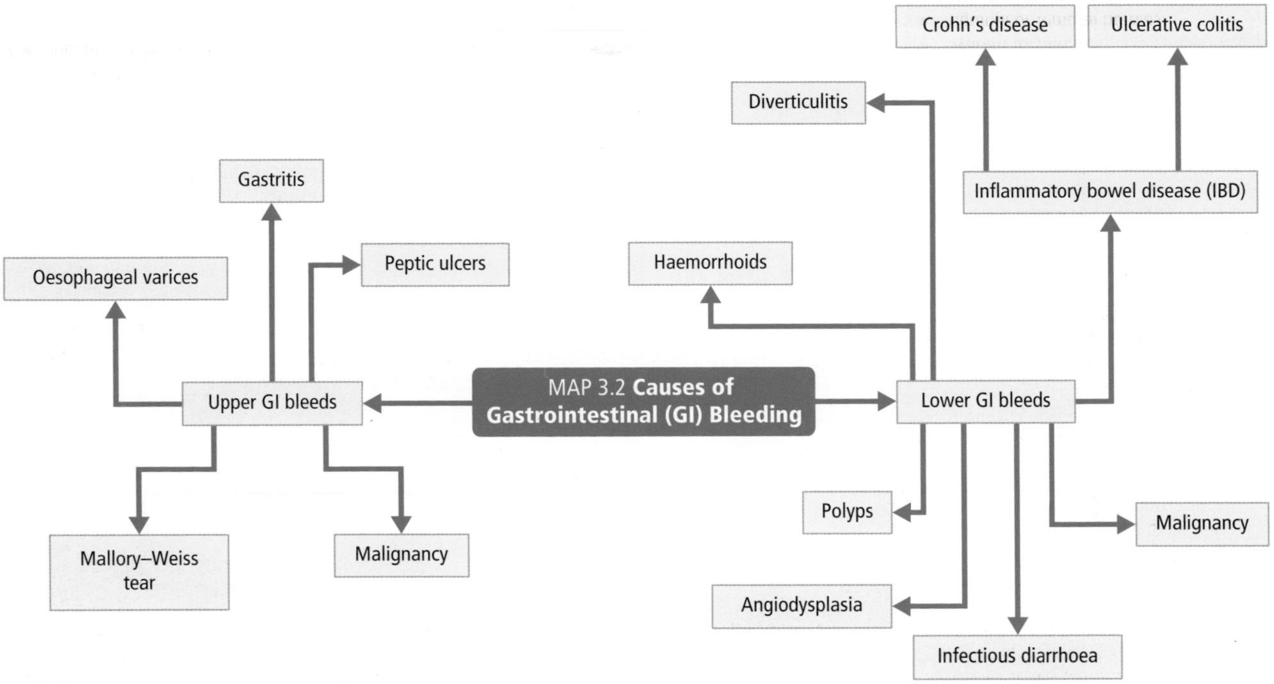

MAP 3.2 **Causes of Gastrointestinal (GI) Bleeding**

Upper GI bleeds
- Peptic ulcers
- Gastritis
- Malignancy
- Oesophageal varices
- Mallory–Weiss tear

Lower GI bleeds
- Inflammatory bowel disease (IBD)
  - Ulcerative colitis
  - Crohn's disease
- Malignancy
- Diverticulitis
- Haemorrhoids
- Polyps
- Infectious diarrhoea
- Angiodysplasia

Map 3.2 Causes of Gastrointestinal (GI) Bleeding

37   **The Gastrointestinal System**

GASTRITIS

What is gastritis?

This is inflammation of the stomach lining. Gastritis may be acute or chronic.

- Acute gastritis, caused by:
  - Stress.
  - NSAIDs.
  - Uraemia.
  - Burns: Curling's ulcer.
  - Alcohol.
- Chronic gastritis:
  - Type A:
    - Autoimmune: autoantibodies are present to parietal cells.
    - Presents with pernicious anaemia.
    - Occurs in the fundus or body of the stomach.
  - Type B:
    - Most common.
    - Associated with *Helicobacter pylori* infection.

Investigate for *H. pylori* infection:

- Bloods: anaemia and *H. pylori*.
- Urinalysis.
- Blood test – measures antibodies to *H. pylori*.
- Carbon isotope–urea breath test.
- Endoscopy with biopsy of stomach lining.
- Stool microscopy and culture – may detect trace amounts of *H. pylori*.

Treatment

- Triple therapy to eradicate *H. pylori*: proton pump inhibitor (PPI), with amoxicillin 1 g and clarithromycin 500 mg or metronidazole 400 mg and clarithromycin 250 mg, taken twice daily.
- Step-wise approach to treating gastritis:
  - Mild – antacids or H_2 receptor antagonists.
  - Moderate/severe – PPI.

Complications

- Peptic ulcers, anaemia (from bleeding ulcers), stricture formation, mucosa-associated lymphoid tissue (MALT) lymphoma.

IRRITABLE BOWEL SYNDROME (IBS)

What is IBS?

This is a common functional disorder of the bowel.

Signs and symptoms

Recurrent abdominal pain, which improves with defaecation; there is a change in bowel habit, i.e. increased or decreased frequency.

Investigations

This is a clinical diagnosis.

Treatment

- Conservative: education and avoidance of triggering factors, e.g. decrease stress.
- Medical: depends on symptoms; antimuscarinics, laxatives, stool softeners, antispasmodics and antidepressants may play a role.

Complications

- Depression and anxiety.

MAP 3.3 Causes of Gastrointestinal (GI) Inflammation

APPENDICITIS
What is appendicitis?
This is inflammation of the appendix that presents with pain that can originate in the umbilical area before migrating to the right iliac fossa.

Investigations
Diagnosis is clinical:
- Bloods: FBC, U&Es, CRP.
- Ultrasound.
- Pregnancy test in females of child bearing age to rule out ectopic pregnancy.

Treatment
- Surgical excision.

Complications
- Peritonitis.

Inflammatory bowel disease (IBD) *(Continued)*

Continued overleaf

Map 3.3 Causes of Gastrointestinal (GI) Inflammation

Map 3.3 Causes of Gastrointestinal (GI) Inflammation

Inflammatory bowel disease (IBD) (Continued)

ULCERATIVE COLITIS
What is ulcerative colitis?
This is a relapsing remitting autoimmune condition that is not associated with granulomas. It affects the colon and rarely the terminal ileum (backwash ileitis).

Signs and symptoms
Remember the **5Ps**:
- **P**yrexia.
- **P**seudopolyps.
- lead **P**ipe radiological appearances.
- **P**oo (bloody diarrhoea).
- **P**roctitis.

Investigations
- These are the same as Crohn's disease.

Treatment
- Conservative: patient education; smoking has been shown to be protective but is not advised.
- Medical: corticosteroids, 5-aminosalicylic acid (5-ASA) analogues (sulfasalazine), mesalazine, 6-mercaptopurine, azathioprine.
- Surgical: colectomy.

Complications
- Toxic megacolon, increased incidence of colon cancer, primary sclerosing cholangitis and osteoporosis (from steroid use).

CROHN'S DISEASE
What is Crohn's disease?
This is a disordered response to intestinal bacteria with transmural inflammation. It may affect any part of the gastrointestinal tract but often targets the terminal ileum. It is associated with granuloma formation.

Signs and symptoms
- Weight loss, abdominal pain (with palpable mass), diarrhoea, fever, skip lesions, clubbing, cobblestone mucosa, fistula formation, fissure formation and linear ulceration.

Investigations
- Bloods: FBC and platelets, U&Es, LFTs and albumin, ESR and CRP.
- Colonoscopy (with biopsy): diagnostic.
- Radiology: small bowel follow through (diagnostic) and abdominal X-ray (for toxic megacolon and excluding perforation).

Treatment
- Conservative: smoking cessation, low residue diet may be encouraged but usually diet is normal.
- Medical: corticosteroids, infliximab, 5-ASA analogues (sulfasalazine), azathioprine, methotrexate.
- Surgical: remove strictured or obstructed region of bowel.

Complications
- Stricture formation, fistula formation, obstruction, pyoderma gangrenosum, anaemia and osteoporosis.

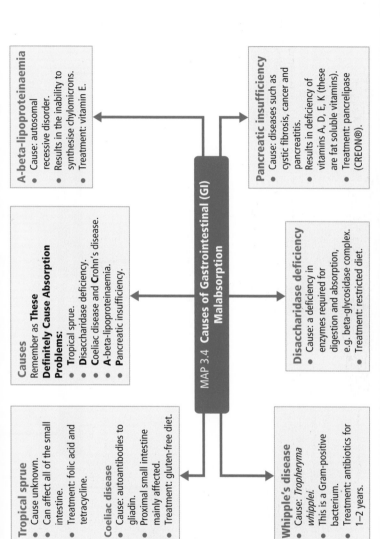

Tropical sprue

- Cause unknown.
- Can affect all of the small intestine.
- Treatment: folic acid and tetracycline.

Coeliac disease

- Cause: autoantibodies to gliadin.
- Proximal small intestine mainly affected.
- Treatment: gluten-free diet.

Whipple's disease

- Cause: *Tropheryma whipplei*.
- This is a Gram-positive bacterium.
- Treatment: antibiotics for 1–2 years.

Causes

Remember as These
**Definitely Cause Absorption
Problems:**

- **T**ropical sprue.
- **D**isaccharidase deficiency.
- **C**oeliac disease and **C**rohn's disease.
- **A**-beta-lipoproteinaemia.
- **P**ancreatic insufficiency.

MAP 3.4 **Causes of Gastrointestinal (GI) Malabsorption**

Disaccharidase deficiency

- Cause: a deficiency in enzymes required for digestion and absorption, e.g. beta-glycosidase complex.
- Treatment: restricted diet.

A-beta-lipoproteinaemia

- Cause: autosomal recessive disorder.
- Results in the inability to synthesise chylomicrons.
- Treatment: vitamin E.

Pancreatic insufficiency

- Cause: diseases such as cystic fibrosis, cancer and pancreatitis.
- Results in deficiency of vitamins A, D, E, K (these are fat soluble vitamins).
- Treatment: pancrelipase (CREON®).

Map 3.4 Causes of Gastrointestinal (GI) Malabsorption

Map 3.5 Gastro-Oesophageal Reflux Disease (GORD)

What is GORD?

This is abnormal reflux where acid from the stomach refluxes into the oesophagus subsequently damaging the squamous oesophageal lining, causing discomfort.

Signs and symptoms

- Heartburn – pain is worse in certain positions, e.g. lying down/stooping and is worse after heavy meals.
- Acid taste in mouth.
  - Regurgitation.
- Water brash (excess salivation).
- Dysphagia.
- Nocturnal asthma/chronic cough.
- Laryngitis.

Causes

- Genetic inheritance of angle of lower oesophageal sphincter.
- Oesophagitis.
- Sliding hiatus hernia.
- Rolling hiatus hernia.

Risk factors

- Smoking.
- Excessive alcohol.
- Excessive coffee.
- Obesity.
- Pregnancy.
- Drugs, e.g. calcium channel blockers, antimuscarinics and tricyclic antidepressants.

Investigations

Age dependent:
- If the patient is <55 years old:
  - Proceed to treatment unless they have ALARM symptoms, e.g. unintentional weight loss, dysphagia, haematemesis, melaena and anorexia.
- If >55 years old:
  - Send patient to endoscopy: diagnostic and allows for biopsy.
  - 24-h pH monitoring.

MAP 3.5 **Gastro-Oesophageal Reflux Disease (GORD)**

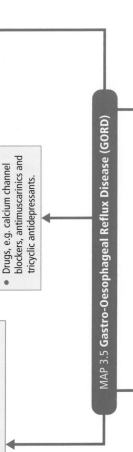

Treatment

- Conservative: education, weight loss, raising head of bed at night and avoidance of precipitating factors, e.g. smoking, large meals.
- Medical:
  - Antacids, e.g. aluminium hydroxide.
  - H_2 receptor antagonists, e.g. ranitidine.
  - Proton pump inhibitors, e.g. omeprazole.
- Surgical: Nissen's fundoplication.

Complications: Barrett's oesophagus
What is Barrett's oesophagus?

This is metaplasia of the normal squamous epithelium of the lower oesophagus to columnar epithelium. This occurs in patients who suffer with GORD for several years. It is a premalignant lesion.

Investigations

- Endoscopy with biopsy in all 4 quadrants.

Treatment

- HALO® system radiofrequency ablation or mucosal resection for highly dysplastic lesions.

Complications

- Adenocarcinoma of the oesophagus.

Map 3.5 Gastro-Oesophageal Reflux Disease (GORD)

What is jaundice?

Jaundice, also known as icterus, is the yellow discolouration of mucous membranes, sclera and skin. This happens due to the accumulation of bilirubin. Jaundice may be seen at a bilirubin concentration >2.5–3.0 mg/dL (42.8–51.3 mmol/L).

Causes

The causes of jaundice may be split into 3 categories (see Table below):

1 Prehepatic jaundice.
2 Intrahepatic jaundice.
3 Posthepatic jaundice.

Treatment

Treat the underlying cause.

Complications

- Liver failure.
- Renal failure.
- Sepsis.
- Pancreatitis.
- Biliary cirrhosis
- Cholangitis
- Kernicterus (a serious complication of jaundice in neonates).

Investigations

You must determine underlying cause.
Use these tests to determine the type of jaundice:

- Appearance of urine and stool.
- LFTs.
- Bilirubin levels.
- Alkaline phosphatase levels.

The different blood results for different types of jaundice:

Investigations	Prehepatic jaundice	Intrahepatic jaundice	Posthepatic jaundice
Appearance of urine	Normal	Dark	Dark
Appearance of stool	Normal	Pale	Pale
Conjugated bilirubin	Normal	↑	↑
Unconjugated bilirubin	Normal or ↑	↑	Normal
Total bilirubin	Normal or ↑	↑	↑
Alkaline phosphatase	Normal	↑	↑

MAP 3.6 Jaundice

The causes of different types of jaundice

Prehepatic jaundice	Intrahepatic jaundice	Posthepatic jaundice
Crigler–Najjar syndrome	Viral and drug induced hepatitis	Gallstones in common bile duct
Gilbert's syndrome	Alcoholic liver disease	Pancreatic cancer
Haemolysis, e.g. thalassaemia, sickle cell anaemia	Hepatic cirrhosis	Schistosomiasis
Drugs, e.g. rifampicin	Primary biliary cirrhosis	Biliary atresia
Malaria	Leptospirosis	Cholangiocarcinoma
Haemolytic uraemic syndrome	Physiological neonatal jaundice	Mirizzi's syndrome

Map 3.6 Jaundice

Map 3.7 Hepatitis Virus

HEPATITIS A (HAV)

What is HAV?

It is a RNA picornavirus.

Transmission

Faecal–oral transmission, associated with contaminated shellfish. The virus passes into bile after replication within liver cells. The immune system is activated by this process and leads to necrosis predominantly in zone 3 of the hepatic lobule.

Incubation period

- 2–3 weeks.

Investigations

- Anti-HAV IgM in serum.

Treatment

- Conservative: vaccine for travellers to endemic areas.
- Medical: supportive since HAV is often self-resolving.

Complications

- Rarely acute liver failure.

HEPATITIS B (HBV)

What is HBV?

A partially stranded, enveloped DNA virus. It has an e-antigen that indicates increased infectivity.

Transmission

- Vertical transmission.
- Contaminated needles.
- Infected blood products.
- Sexual intercourse.

Incubation period

- 1–5 months.

Investigations

HBV DNA in serum, HBsAg, HBeAg, anti-HBc; HBsAg presents on histology with a 'ground glass' appearance.

Treatment

- Conservative: education and prevention of disease; vaccine for at-risk groups, e.g. health workers.
- Medical: antiviral medications, e.g. pegylated alpha-2a interferon, adefovir, entecavir, lamivudine, tenofovir, telbivudine.

Complications

- Hepatic cirrhosis, hepatocellular carcinoma (HCC), fulminant hepatitis B.

MAP 3.7 **Hepatitis Virus**

HEPATITIS C (HCV)
What is HCV?
It is a single stranded, enveloped RNA virus and a member of the flavivirus family.

Transmission
- Vertical transmission (occasionally).
- Contaminated needles.
- Infected blood products.

Incubation period
- Intermediate (6–9 weeks).

Investigations
- Antibody to HCV in the serum.

Treatment
- Conservative: education and prevention of disease.
- Medical: antiviral medications, e.g. pegylated alpha-2a interferon, ribavirin, taribavirin, telaprevir.

Complications
- Hepatic cirrhosis, HCC, liver failure.

HEPATITIS D (HDV)
What is HDV?
It is a single stranded defective RNA virus that co-infects with hepatitis B virus. Co-infectivity with HDV leads to an increased chance of liver failure.

Transmission
- Contaminated needles.
- Infected blood products.
- Sexual intercourse (rare).

Incubation period
- 1–5 months.

Investigations
- Serum IgM anti-D.

Treatment
- Pegylated alpha-2a interferon.

Complications
- Hepatic cirrhosis, HCC.

Hepatitis E (HEV)
What is HEV?
It is a single stranded RNA virus.

Transmission
- Faecal–oral transmission, associated with contaminated water.

Incubation period
- 2–3 weeks.

Investigations
- IgG and IgM anti-HEV.

Treatment
- Usually self-limiting.

Complications
- High mortality of pregnant women (~20%).

Map 3.7 Hepatitis Virus

What is CRC?

This is cancer of the colon and rectum and is the third most common malignancy.
Usually adenocarcinoma on histology.

Signs and symptoms

- Abdominal pain.
- Unintentional weight loss.
- Altered bowel habit.
- Faecal occult blood.
- Anaemia.
- Fatigue.

Causes

Multifactorial and often unknown. There are risk factors that may predispose an
individual to develop CRC (see risk factor box).

Investigations

- Bowel Cancer Screening Programme: faecal occult blood test in men and women
  aged 60–69 years.
- Bloods: FBC for iron deficiency anaemia and carcinoembryonic antigen (CEA)
  tumour marker.
- Endoscopy: colonoscopy/sigmoidoscopy.
- Imaging: double contrast barium enema study 'apple core' sign; virtual colonoscopy.

Treatment

Depends on the extent of disease. This is assessed using Dukes staging system or
TNM system.

- Conservative: patient education and referral to Macmillan nurses.

Risk factors

- Smoking.
- Increased age.
- Family history of CRC.
- Inflammatory bowel disease (IBD).
- *Streptococcus bovis* bacteraemia.
- Congenital polyposis syndromes:
  ○ Juvenile polyposis syndrome:
    – Autosomal dominant but it may occur spontaneously.
    – Not malignant.
  ○ Peutz–Jeghers syndrome:
    – Autosomal dominant.
    – Increases risk of CRC.
    – Melanosis is present on the oral mucosa.
- Genetic predisposition:
  ○ Familial adenomatous polyposis (FAP):
    – Autosomal dominant.
    – Mutation of *APC* gene on chromosome 5.
    – 100% lead to CRC.
  ○ Hereditary nonpolyposis colorectal cancer (HNPCC):
    – Autosomal dominant.
    – Mutation of DNA mismatch repair gene.

- Medical: chemotherapy (oxaliplatin, folinic acid and 5-fluorouracil is the most common regime); radiotherapy may also be used.
- Surgery: surgical resection is usually treatment of choice.

Complications
- Obstruction and metastasis.

MAP 3.8 Colorectal Cancer (CRC)

TNM system

T – Carcinoma *in situ*
T1 – Submucosa invaded
T2 – Muscularis mucosa invaded
T3 – Tumour has invaded subserosa but other organs have not been penetrated
T4 – Adjacent organs invaded

N1 – Metastatic spread to 1–3 regional lymph nodes
N2 – Metastatic spread to ≥4 regional lymph nodes

M0 – No distant metastases present
M1 – Distant metastases present

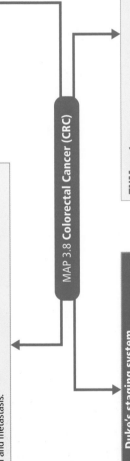

Duke's staging system		
Stage	**Description**	**5-year survival**
A	Confined to muscularis mucosa	90%
B	Extends through muscularis mucosa	65%
C	Lymph node involvement	30%
D	Distant metastases	<10%

Map 3.8 Colorectal Cancer (CRC)

Map 3.9 Pancreatitis

MAP 3.9 Pancreatitis

ACUTE PANCREATITIS
What is acute pancreatitis?
This is inflammation of the pancreatic parenchyma, with biochemical associations of increased amylase and raised lipase enzymes on blood test.

Signs and symptoms
Remember these as **PAN:**
- Epigastric **P**ain that radiates to the back.
- **A**norexia.
- **N**ausea and vomiting.
- Grey Turner's sign: flank bruising.
- Cullen's sign: periumbilical bruising.

Causes
Remember these as **GET SMASHED:**
- **G**allstones.
- **E**thanol.
- **T**rauma.

CHRONIC PANCREATITIS
What is chronic pancreatitis?
This is where the structural integrity of the pancreas is permanently altered as a direct result of chronic inflammation.

Signs and symptoms
Pain! The pain is:
- Epigastric in origin.
- Recurrent.
- Radiates to the back.
- Relieved by sitting forward.
- Worse when eating/drinking heavily.

Causes
Remember these as **CAMP:**
- **C**ystic fibrosis.
- **A**lcohol.
- **M**alnourishment.
- **P**ancreatic duct obstruction.

- Scorpion sting (*Tityus trinitatis*).
- Mumps.
- Autoimmune disease.
- Steroids.
- **H**yperlipidaemia/**H**ypercalcaemia.
- Endoscopic retrograde cholangiopancreatography (ERCP).
- Drugs, e.g. azathioprine.

Investigations
- Raised serum amylase and lipase.
- Detect cause, e.g. ultrasound scan to detect presence of gallstones.
- CT scan to rule out complications (not within <72 h of acute presentation unless clinically indicated).

Treatment
- This is usually symptomatic relief. Keep 'nil by mouth' (NBM), IV fluids and analgesia, e.g. tramadol
- Treat underlying causes, e.g. ERCP to remove gallstones.

Complications
Remember these as **HDAMN**:
- **H**aemorrhage.
- **D**isseminated intravascular coagulation (DIC).
- **A**cute respiratory distress syndrome (ARDS).
- **M**ultiorgan failure.
- **N**ecrosis.

Investigations
- Decreased faecal elastase.
- CT scan: shows calcification (may also be seen on abdominal X-ray).
- Magnetic resonance cholangiopancreatography (MRCP).

Treatment
- Conservative: alcohol cessation.
- Medical: analgesia, e.g. tramadol and pancreatic enzyme replacement therapy; start insulin therapy if diabetes has developed.

Complications
Remember these as **PODS**:
- **P**seudocysts.
- **O**bstruction (pancreatic).
- **D**iabetes mellitus.
- **S**teatorrhoea.

Map 3.9 Pancreatitis

Table 3.1 Microbiology of the Gastrointestinal (GI) Tract

TABLE 3.1 Microbiology of the Gastrointestinal (GI) Tract

Organism	Illness caused	Other
Vibrio vulnificus	Food poisoning	Found in seafood; Gram-negative bacterium
Bacillus cereus	Food poisoning	Found in reheated rice; Gram-positive bacterium
Staphylococcus aureus	Food poisoning	Found in contaminated meat and mayonnaise; Gram-positive bacterium
Clostridium botulinum	Food poisoning	Found in poorly canned foods; Gram-positive bacterium
Escherichia coli O157:H7	Food poisoning and diarrhoea	Found in meat that is undercooked; enteropathogenic *E.coli* causes diarrhoea in children; also causes haemolytic uraemic syndrome (HUS); Gram-negative bacterium
Campylobacter jejuni	Bloody diarrhoea	Found in animal faeces and poultry; it is associated with Guillain–Barré syndrome, which is an ascending paralysis; Gram-negative bacterium
Salmonella	Bloody diarrhoea	Found in contaminated food; Gram-negative bacterium
Shigella	Bloody diarrhoea	Produces shiga toxin; Gram-negative bacterium
Yersinia enterocolitica	Bloody diarrhoea	Associated with outbreaks in nurseries; Gram-negative bacterium
Enterotoxic *Escherichia coli*	Traveller's diarrhoea	Traveller's diarrhoea is usually self-limiting; Gram-negative bacterium
Vibrio cholerae	Rice water diarrhoea	Produces cholera toxin; Gram-negative bacterium
Cryptosporidium	Cryptosporidiosis	Associated with AIDS patients; protozoon
Norwalk virus	Gastroenteritis	Most common viral cause of nausea and vomiting
Helicobacter pylori	Risk factors for peptic ulcers, gastritis and gastric adenocarcinoma	Produces urease; treat with 'triple therapy', i.e. a proton pump inhibitor (PPI) with either clarithromycin and amoxicillin or clarithromycin and metronidazole; Gram-negative bacterium
Toxoplasma gondii	Toxoplasmosis	Cysts are found in meat or cat faeces; causes brain abscesses in AIDS patients; protozoon
Taenia solium	Intestinal tapeworms	Found in undercooked pork; cestode

Figure 4.1 Nephron Physiology

FIGURE 4.1 Nephron Physiology

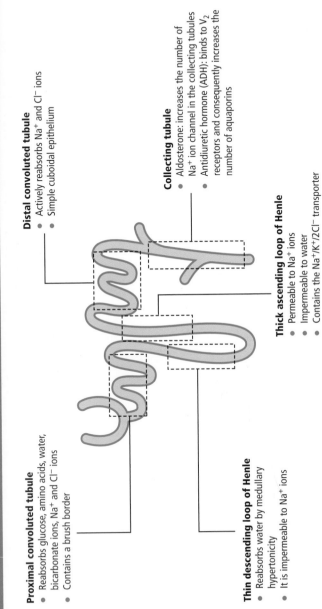

Proximal convoluted tubule
- Reabsorbs glucose, amino acids, water, bicarbonate ions, Na^+ and Cl^- ions
- Contains a brush border

Distal convoluted tubule
- Actively reabsorbs Na^+ and Cl^- ions
- Simple cuboidal epithelium

Collecting tubule
- Aldosterone: increases the number of Na^+ ion channel in the collecting tubules
- Antidiuretic hormone (ADH): binds to V_2 receptors and consequently increases the number of aquaporins

Thin descending loop of Henle
- Reabsorbs water by medullary hypertonicity
- It is impermeable to Na^+ ions

Thick ascending loop of Henle
- Permeable to Na^+ ions
- Impermeable to water
- Contains the $Na^+/K^+/2Cl^-$ transporter

FIGURE 4.2 **The Renin Angiotensin Aldosterone System (RAAS)**

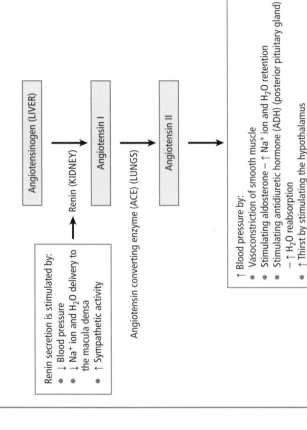

Renin secretion is stimulated by:
- ↓ Blood pressure
- ↓ Na$^+$ ion and H$_2$O delivery to the macula densa
- ↑ Sympathetic activity

Angiotensinogen (LIVER)

→ Renin (KIDNEY)

Angiotensin I

Angiotensin converting enzyme (ACE) (LUNGS)

Angiotensin II

↑ Blood pressure by:
- Vasoconstriction of smooth muscle
- Stimulating aldosterone – ↑ Na$^+$ ion and H$_2$O retention
- Stimulating antidiuretic hormone (ADH) (posterior pituitary gland)
  – ↑ H$_2$O reabsorption
- ↑ Thirst by stimulating the hypothalamus

Figure 4.2 The Renin Angiotensin Aldosterone System (RAAS)

TABLE 4.1 **Diuretics**

Class of diuretic	Example	Mechanism of action	Uses	Side-effects	Contraindications	Drug interactions
Thiazide diuretic	Bendroflumethiazide	Blocks Na$^+$/Cl$^-$ ion symporter in the distal convoluted tubule	Hypertension Heart failure Ascites	Hyponatraemia Hypokalaemia Hypercalcaemia Hyperglycaemia Hyperlipidaemia Hyperuricaemia	Gout Liver failure Renal failure May worsen diabetes	Hypokalaemia may increase the risk of digoxin toxicity Decreased lithium excretion
Loop diuretic	Furosemide	Blocks Na$^+$/K$^+$/2Cl$^-$ co-transporter in the ascending loop of Henle	Heart failure (symptomatic treatment of oedema) Severe hypercalcaemia	Hyponatraemia Hypokalaemia Hypocalcaemia Ototoxicity	Renal failure	Hypokalaemia may increase the risk of digoxin toxicity Decreased lithium excretion
K$^+$ sparing diuretic	Spironolactone	Aldosterone receptor antagonist	Heart failure (in combination with furosemide) Oedema Ascites Refractory hypertension Conn's syndrome	Hyperkalaemia Gynaecomastia (alternatively, eplerenone can be given as a more selective aldosterone antagonist)	Addison's disease Hyperkalaemia	Decreased lithium excretion
Osmotic diuretic	Mannitol	Increases plasma osmolarity	Cerebral oedema Rhabdomyolysis Haemolysis	Fever Hyponatraemia	Heart failure	Increases levels of tobramycin

Table 4.1 Diuretics

Treatment

- Conservative: prevent cause, e.g. low calcium diet. Education about risk factors.
- Medical:

Symptom	Treatment
Pain	Analgesia and tamsulosin
Dehydration	IV and oral fluids
Nausea/vomiting	Antiemetics
↑ Calcium	Low calcium diet and stop thiazide diuretics if possible
↑ Oxalate	Low oxalate diet
↑ Uric acid	Allopurinol

- Radiology:
  - Nephrostomy insertion.
  - Antegrade ureteric stent insertion.
- Surgical:
  - Antegrade or retrograde removal of large stones or staghorn calculus.
  - Extracorporeal shock wave lithotripsy (ESWL) for the treatment of larger stones (>0.5 cm).

Causes

- Idiopathic.
- Hypercalcaemia.
- Hyperuricaemia.
- Hyperoxaluria.
- Recurrent UTI.
- Drugs, e.g. loop diuretics.
- Hereditary conditions increase risk, e.g. polycystic kidney disease.

MAP 4.1 Renal Calculi

What are renal calculi?

These are stones that form within the renal tract. Most stones are made from calcium (radiopaque), but others are made from struvite (staghorn calculus) and uric acid crystals (radiolucent).

Signs and symptoms

- Asymptomatic.
- Pain (suprapubic and loin pain that may radiate to the genital region).
- Dysuria.
- Urinary tract infection (UTI).
- Haematuria.

Complications

- Recurrent UTI.
- Recurrent calculi.
- Obstruction.
- Trauma to ureter/ureteric stricture.

Investigations

- 24-h urine analysis: assess levels of calcium, uric acid, oxalate and citrate.
- CT kidney, ureter, bladder (KUB): for radiopaque stones.
- Ultrasound and IVU can also be utilised.
- Chemical analysis of stone composition.

Map 4.1 Renal Calculi

Map 4.2 Urinary Tract Infection (UTI)

What is a UTI?

This is an infection of the urinary tract with typical signs and symptoms. It may be classified as either a lower or upper (acute pyelonephritis) UTI.

Signs and symptoms of lower UTI

- Dysuria.
- Frequency.
- Urgency.
- Suprapubic pain.

Signs and symptoms of upper UTI

- Fever/chills.
- Flank pain.
- Haematuria.

Risk factors

- Female gender.
- Sexual intercourse.
- Catheterisation.
- Pregnancy.
- Menopause.
- Diabetes.
- Genitourinary malformation.
- Immunosuppression.
- Urinary tract obstruction, e.g. stones.

Pathophysiology

The urinary system has many defences to prevent UTI such as:

- Micturition.
- Urine: osmolarity, pH and organic acids are antibacterial.
- Secreted factors:
  - Tamm–Horsfall protein: binds bacteria nonspecifically; produced by cells of the thick ascending loop of Henle; mutations in the gene that codes for this protein are associated with progressive renal failure and medullary cysts.
  - IgA: against specific bacteria.
  - Lactoferrin: hoovers up free iron.
- Mucosal defences: mucopolysaccharides coat the mucosal surfaces of the bladder.
- If these defence mechanisms are overcome by bacterial virulence factors then the patient is prone to developing a UTI. Some virulence factors worth noting are:
- For uropathogenic *E. coli* (UPEC):
  - Type 1 fimbriae: binds to mannose residues; associated with cystitis.
  - Type P fimbriae: binds to glycolipid residues; associated with pyelonephritis.
  - Bacterial capsule: aka antigen K, resists phagocytosis; associated with pyelonephritis.
- For *Proteus mirabilis*:
  - Produces urease.
  - Increases pH of urine.
  - *Proteus mirabilis* is associated with staghorn calculi.

MAP 4.2 Urinary Tract Infection (UTI)

Causative organisms

- *Escherichia coli*: leading cause of UTI in the community and also nosocomial infection. Metallic sheen on eosin methylene blue (EMB).
- *Staphylococcus saprophyticus*: 2nd leading cause in sexually active females.
- *Klebsiella pneumoniae*: 3rd leading cause. Viscous colonies.
- *Proteus mirabilis*: produces urease. Gram-negative bacterium.
- *Pseudomonas aeruginosa*: bile green pigment and fruity odour. Usually nosocomial and drug resistant.
- Adenovirus: haemorrhagic cystitis.
- BK and JC viruses: associated with graft failure after transplant.
- *Schistosoma haematobium*: parasitic infection.

Investigations

- Urine dipstick: positive for leucocytes and nitrites.
- Urine culture: for diagnosis for causative organism (>10^5 organisms per mL of midstream urine).
- Radiology: consider ultrasound scan or cystoscopy if UTI occurs in children, in men or if UTI is recurrent.

Treatment

- Conservative: education about the condition and avoidance of predisposing risk factors.
- Medical: trimethoprim twice daily. Consider prophylactic antibiotics if UTI is recurrent.
- If recurrent, i.e. >4 UTIs per year, seek to exclude anatomical variant or abnormality of the renal tract.

Complications

- Pyelonephritis.
- Renal failure.
- Sepsis.

Map 4.2 Urinary Tract Infection (UTI)

Map 4.3 Renal Cancers

MAP 4.3 Renal Cancers

RENAL CELL CARCINOMA (RCC)

What is RCC?

This is an adenocarcinoma originating from the cells that line the proximal convoluted tubule.

Risk factors

- Male.
- Age 50–70 years.
- Smoking.
- Obesity.
- Mutation of the Von Hippel–Lindau tumour suppressor gene on chromosome 3.

Signs and symptoms

- Unintentional weight loss.
- Loin pain.
- Haematuria.
- Palpable mass.
- Fever.
- Hypertension.

TRANSITIONAL CELL CARCINOMA (TCC)

What is TCC?

This is a cancer that arises from transitional urothelium. It is more common in men.

Risk factors

Remember these as **CAPS**:

- **C**yclophosphamide.
- **A**niline dyes.
- **P**henacetin.
- **S**moking.

Signs and symptoms

Depends on the location of the cancer but is usually associated with painless haematuria and lower urinary tract symptoms, e.g. frequency and urgency.

Paraneoplastic syndromes involved

- Secretion of adrenocorticotrophic hormone (ACTH): may produce symptoms of hypercalcaemia.
- Secretion of erythropoietin (EPO): may produce symptoms of polycythaemia.

Investigations

- Radiology (ultrasound scan, CT scan, MRI scan).

Treatment

- Conservative: patient education. Supportive, counselling and monitoring of psychological wellbeing (depression). Refer patients to Macmillan nurses.
- Medical: interferon alpha, sunitinib, sorafenib, bevacizumab.
- Surgical: partial or total nephrectomy is the treatment of choice; radiofrequency ablation may be considered.

Complications

- Metastasis: to brain, bone, lung, liver, adrenal glands and lymph nodes.
- Hypercalcaemia.
- Hypertension.
- Polycythaemia.

Investigations

- Cystoscopy and ureteroscopy with biopsy.
- Retrograde pyelography.
- CT scan.
- MRI scan.

Treatment

- Conservative: supportive counselling and monitoring of psychological wellbeing (depression). Refer patients to Macmillan nurses.
- Medical: mitomycin, GC regimen (gemcitabine and cisplatin) or MVAC regimen (methotrexate, vinblastine, adriamycin and cisplatin).
- Surgical: nephroureterectomy, cystectomy; radiofrequency ablation may be considered.

Complications

- Metastasis, usually to bone.

Map 4.4 Kidney Injury

MAP 4.4 Kidney Injury

ACUTE KIDNEY INJURY (AKI)

What is AKI?

This is when the kidney fails over a short time period (days to weeks) and is characterised by a rapid fall in glomerular filtration rate (GFR) and an increase in creatinine and urea levels. It may be reversible. AKI may be subdivided into prerenal, intrinsic renal and postrenal failure and these have many different causes.

Causes

Prerenal	Intrinsic	Postrenal
Hypovolaemia <ul><li>Haemorrhage</li><li>Burns</li><li>Diuretic use</li></ul>	Glomerular disease <ul><li>Glomerulonephritis</li><li>Vasculitis</li><li>Immune complex disease, e.g. systemic lupus erythematosus (SLE)</li></ul>	Obstruction of the ureter <ul><li>Stones</li><li>Tumour</li></ul>
Shock <ul><li>Sepsis</li><li>Cardiogenic</li></ul>	Vascular lesions <ul><li>Bilateral renal artery stenosis</li><li>Microangiopathy</li><li>Malignant hypertension</li></ul>	Obstruction of the bladder neck <ul><li>Stones</li><li>Tumour</li><li>Benign prostatic hypertrophy</li><li>Prostate cancer</li></ul>
Hypoperfusion <ul><li>Hepatorenal syndrome</li><li>NSAID use</li></ul>	Tubulointerstitial disease <ul><li>Acute tubular necrosis</li><li>Acute tubulointerstitial nephritis</li></ul>	Obstruction of the urethra <ul><li>Tumour</li><li>Stricture</li></ul>

CHRONIC KIDNEY INJURY (CKI)

What is CKI?

This is well-established renal impairment and is irreversible. Renal function progressively worsens with time. Without treatment the patient will eventually develop end-stage kidney disease (ESKD).

Causes

- Any renal disease may lead to CKI.
- Glomerulonephritis.
- Hypertension.
- Diabetes mellitus.
- Malignancy.
- Anatomical abnormality of the renal tract.
- Hereditary disease, e.g. polycystic kidney disease.

Signs and symptoms

Oliguria/anuria/polyuria, nausea and vomiting, confusion, hypertension, oedema (peripheral and pulmonary), fatigue, metallic taste in mouth, unintentional weight loss, itchy skin, skin pigmentation, Kaussmaul breathing (metabolic acidosis), anaemia.

• Angiotensin converting enzyme (ACE) inhibitor use	• Multiple myeloma • Nephrotoxic drugs
Oedematous conditions • Heart failure • Nephrotic syndrome	

Signs and symptoms

Oliguria/anuria, nausea and vomiting, confusion, hypertension, abdominal/flank pain, signs of fluid overload, e.g. ↑ jugular venous pressure (JVP).

Investigations

- GFR.
- Bloods: FBC and platelets, U&Es, creatinine, calcium and phosphate levels, ESR, CRP, immunology, virology.
- Urinalysis: blood, protein, glucose, leucocytes and nitrites, Bence Jones protein.
- Imaging: ultrasound scan.

Treatment

- Maintain renal blood flow and fluid balance.
- Monitor electrolytes.
- Treat underlying cause; classify AKI with **RIFLE** criteria (**R**isk, **I**njury, **F**ailure, **L**oss, **E**nd-stage renal disease).
- Stop all nephrotoxic drugs.

Complications

- Metabolic acidosis.
- Hyperkalaemia.
- Hyperphosphataemia.
- Pulmonary oedema.

Investigations

- GFR.
- Bloods: FBC, U&Es, creatinine, calcium and phosphate levels, ESR, CRP, immunology, virology.
- Urinalysis: blood, protein, glucose, leucocytes and nitrites; Bence Jones proteinuria (multiple myeloma).
- Imaging: ultrasound scan.
- Renal biopsy.

Treatment

- Conservative: smoking cessation, low salt diet, maintain psychological wellbeing.
- Medical:
  ○ Treat underlying cause and complications.
  ○ Control blood pressure.
  ○ Treat anaemia.
  ○ Treat acidosis (with sodium bicarbonate).
  ○ Treat hyperphosphataemia (with phosphate binders).
- Surgical: dialysis (haemodialysis or peritoneal dialysis), renal transplantation.

Complications

- Anaemia.
- Hypertension.
- Renal bone disease.
- Metabolic acidosis.
- Stroke.
- Peripheral nerve damage.
- Carpal tunnel syndrome.
- Oedematous states.
- Depression.

Map 4.5 Nephritic vs. Nephrotic Syndrome

MAP 4.5 **Nephritic vs. Nephrotic Syndrome**

NEPHRITIC SYNDROME

What is nephritic syndrome?

This is a group of signs of varying diseases.

Signs

Remember these as **PHARAOH**:

- **P**roteinuria.
- **H**aematuria.
- **A**zotaemia.
- **R**ed blood cell casts.
- **A**ntistreptolysin O titres.
- **O**liguria.
- **H**ypertension.

Causes

These may be split broadly into 2 categories: focal proliferative and diffuse proliferative causes.

Focal proliferative	Diffuse proliferative
IgA nephropathy	Rapidly progressive glomerulonephritis, e.g. Goodpasture's syndrome
Systemic lupus erythematosus (SLE)	SLE
Henoch–Schönlein purpura	Membranoproliferative glomerulonephritis
Alport's syndrome	Cryoglobulinaemia

NEPHROTIC SYNDROME

What is nephrotic syndrome?

This is a group of signs of varying diseases.

Signs

Remember these as **PHHO**:

- **P**roteinuria >3 g daily.
- **H**ypoalbuminaemia <30 g/L.
- **H**yperlipidaemia, occurs because:
  - Hypoproteinaemia stimulates the production of more proteins from the liver, which results in the synthesis of more lipoproteins.
  - Decreased levels of lipoprotein lipase means that lipid catabolism decreases.
- **O**edema.

Causes

- Minimal change disease.
- Focal segmental glomerulosclerosis.
- Membranous glomerulonephritis.
- Diabetic nephropathy.
- Amyloidosis.

Investigations

- Bloods: FBC, WCC and platelets, U&Es, LFTs, creatinine, urea, CRP, ESR, glucose, lipid profile.
- Urinalysis: blood, protein, glucose, leucocytes, nitrites and Bence Jones protein.
- Nephritic screen: serum complement (C3 and C4), antinuclear antibody (ANA), double stranded DNA, antineutrophil cytoplasmic antibody (ANCA), antiglomerular basement membrane (GBM), HIV serology, HBV and HCV serology, blood cultures, Venereal Disease Research Laboratory Test (VDRL) for syphilis.
- Renal biopsy.
- Radiology: ultrasound scan.

Treatment

- Conservative: lifestyle advice, low salt diet.
- Medical: treatment depends on cause:
  - Treat hypertension.
  - Treat proteinuria.
  - Treat hypercholesterolaemia.
  - Give prophylactic anticoagulation therapy.
  - Immunotherapy regimen, e.g. prednisolone, cyclophosphamide and azathioprine.
  - Dialysis if severe.

Complications

- Nephrotic syndrome.
- Chronic glomerulonephritis.
- Heart failure.

- Mesangial proliferative glomerulonephritis.
- SLE.

Investigations

- Bloods: FBC, WCC and platelets, U&Es, LFTs, creatinine, urea, CRP, ESR, glucose, lipid profile.
- Urinalysis: blood, protein, glucose, leucocytes, nitrites and Bence Jones protein.
- Nephritic screen: serum complement (C3 and C4), ANA, dsDNA, ANCA, anti-GBM, HIV serology, HBV and HCV serology, blood cultures, VDRL for syphilis.
- Renal biopsy.
- Radiology: ultrasound scan.

Treatment

- Conservative: lifestyle advice, low salt diet.
- Medical: treatment depends on cause:
  - Treat hypertension.
  - Treat proteinuria.
  - Treat hypercholesterolaemia.
  - Give prophylactic anticoagulation therapy.
  - Immunotherapy regimen, e.g. prednisolone, cyclophosphamide and azathioprine.
  - Dialysis if severe.

Complications

- Hypertension.
- Acute kidney injury.
- Chronic kidney injury.
- Infection.

ADPKD

What is ADPKD?

This is a dominantly inherited polycystic disease found in adults.

Causes

Mutations in the genes encoding a membrane protein called polycystin result in this condition. Two genes code for this protein:

- *PKD1* on chromosome 16 (encodes polycystin 1).
- *PKD2* on chromosome 4 (encodes polycystin 2).

Signs and symptoms

- Pain (due to renal cyst haemorrhage).
- Hypertension.
- Haematuria.
- Palpable bilateral flank masses.
- Hepatomegaly.

Investigations

- Bloods: FBC, U&Es, calcium and phosphate, PTH.
- Urinalysis and culture.
- Imaging: ultrasound scan is diagnostic.
- Genetic screening and monitoring of blood pressure.

Remember cystic disease as CAAR

- **C**ystic renal dysplasia.
- **A**utosomal dominant polycystic kidney disease (ADPKD).
- **A**utosomal recessive polycystic kidney disease (ARPKD).
- Cystic diseases of the **R**enal medulla.

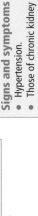

MAP 4.6
Cystic Disease

ARPKD

What is ARPKD?

This is a recessively inherited polycystic disease found in children presenting with varying levels of kidney and liver disease.

Causes

- *PKHD1* on chromosome 6.

Signs and symptoms

- Hypertension.
- Those of chronic kidney injury.
- Chronic respiratory infections.
- Those of portal hypertension: ascites, caput medusae and oesophageal varices.
- Failure to thrive.
- Recurrent UTI.
- Polyuria.

Investigations

- Antenatal screening is diagnostic.
- Bloods: FBC, U&Es, LFTs.
- Urinalysis and culture.
- Imaging: ultrasound scan (shows enlarged kidney with or without oligohydramnios), CT scan, MRI scan.

Treatment

- Conservative: parental and patient support.
- Medical:
  - Ventilation and long-term oxygen therapy.
  - Treat hypertension (angiotensin converting enzyme [ACE] inhibitors).
  - Antibiotics for UTI.
  - Diuretics for fluid overload.
- Surgical:
  - Nephrectomy.
  - Combined renal and liver transplant.

Complications

- Hepatic cysts.
- Congenital hepatic fibrosis.
- Proliferative bile ducts.

Cystic diseases of the renal medulla

Remember **NAMS**:

- **N**ephronophthisis medullary cystic disease.
- **A**cquired cystic disease: usually from dialysis.
- **M**edullary sponge kidney.
- **S**imple cysts.

Treatment

- Conservative: patient support.
- Medical:
  - Treat hypertension.
  - Antibiotic therapy for urinary trait infection (UTI).
- Surgical: cyst decompression.

Complications

- Development of chronic kidney injury.
- Remember **LAMB**:
  - **L**iver cysts.
  - **A**neurysms.
  - **M**itral valve prolapse.
  - **B**erry aneurysm rupture leading to subarachnoid haemorrhage.

Map 4.6 Cystic Disease

Map 4.7 Congenital Kidney Abnormalities

ECTOPIC KIDNEY

What is an ectopic kidney?
This is a congenital abnormality in which the kidney lies above the pelvic brim or within the pelvis.

Signs and symptoms
- Usually asymptomatic.

Causes
- Genetic abnormalities.
- Poor development of the metanephrogenic diverticulum.
- Teratogen exposure.

Investigations
- Ultrasound scan is diagnostic.

Treatment
- None; treat complications should they develop.

Complications
- UTI.
- Renal calculi.

Remember these as HERD
- **H**orseshoe kidney.
- **E**ctopic kidney.
- **R**enal agenesis.
- **D**uplex ureters.

HORSESHOE KIDNEY

What is a horseshoe kidney?
This occurs during development when the lower poles of both kidneys fuse, resulting in the formation of one horseshoe-shaped kidney. This cannot ascend to the normal anatomical position due to the central fused portion catching the inferior mesenteric artery.

Signs and symptoms
- Asymptomatic.
- Recurrent urinary tract infection (UTI).
- Renal calculi.
- Obstructive uropathy.

Causes
- Congenital abnormality.

Investigations
- Ultrasound scan is diagnostic.

Treatment
- Treatment of complications.

Complications
- Susceptible to trauma.
- Renal calculi formation.
- Increased risk of transitional cell carcinoma of the renal pelvis.

MAP 4.7 **Congenital Kidney Abnormalities**

DUPLEX URETERS

What are duplex ureters?

This occurs when the ureteric bud splits during embryonic development and results in the development of 2 ureters, which drain 1 kidney.

Signs and symptoms

- Asymptomatic.
- Recurrent UTI.

Causes

- Splitting of the ureteric bud.

Investigations

- Ultrasound scan and excretory urography is diagnostic.

Treatment

- Treatment of complications.

Complications

- Vesicoureteral reflux.
- Ureterocele.
- UTI.

RENAL AGENESIS

What is renal agenesis?

Bilateral or unilateral absence of the kidney.

Signs and symptoms

Bilateral absence (Potter's syndrome)	Unilateral absence
Low set ears	Hypertension
Limb defects	Increased risk of respiratory infections
Receding chin	Proteinuria
Flat, broad nose	Haematuria

Causes

- Failure of the ureteric bud development.

Investigations

- Antenatal screening.

Treatment

This depends on whether there is bilateral or unilateral absence of the kidney.

Bilateral absence (Potter's syndrome)	Unilateral absence
Neonates usually die a few days after birth. If the baby survives they require chronic peritoneal dialysis	Treatment of hypertension

Complications

- Susceptible to trauma (unilateral).
- Death.

Map 4.7 Congenital Kidney Abnormalities

Map 5.1 Hyperthyroidism

What is hyperthyroidism?

This occurs when there is too much circulating thyroid hormone in the body.
There are many different causes of hyperthyroidism.

Signs and symptoms

- Weight loss.
- Warm skin/heat intolerance.
- Diarrhoea.
- Exophthalmos (Graves' disease).
- Lid lag.
- Palpitations.
- Anxiety.
- Tremor.
- Goitre +/– bruit.
- Brisk reflexes.

MAP 5.1
Hyperthyroidism

Causes

Cause	Comment
Graves' disease	<ul><li>This is the most common cause of hyperthyroidism</li><li>It is an autoimmune condition</li><li>May be distinguished from other causes of hyperthyroidism by ocular changes, e.g. exophthalmos, and other signs, e.g. pretibial myxoedema</li><li>It is associated with other autoimmune conditions such as pernicious anaemia</li></ul>
Toxic multinodular goitre and toxic solitary nodule goitre	<ul><li>This is the second most common cause of hyperthyroidism</li><li>Risk increases with age</li><li>More common in females</li><li>A single nodule is suggestive of thyroid neoplasia</li></ul>
De Quervain's thyroiditis	<ul><li>This is transient hyperthyroidism that develops after a viral infection</li><li>Goitre is often painful</li><li>A period of hypothyroidism may follow</li></ul>

Investigations

- TFTs ($\downarrow$ TSH, $\uparrow$ T3 and $\uparrow$ T4).
- Ultrasound scan of nodules.
- Fine needle aspiration of solitary nodules to exclude malignancy.
- Isotope scan to assess hot and cold thyroid nodules.

Treatment

- Conservative: patient education, smoking cessation.
- Medical:

Symptomatic control	Palpitations and tremor: beta-blockers Eye symptoms: eye drops for lubrication
Antithyroid medication	Carbimazole Propylthiouracil Side-effects: agranulocytosis (monitor patient's bloods carefully)
Radioactive iodine ablation	Definitive treatment; patients must be euthyroid before commencing treatment

- Surgical: subtotal thyroidectomy; patients must be euthyroid before the procedure. Give the patient potassium iodide before surgery since it decreases thyroid gland vascularity.

Complications

- Atrial fibrillation.
- High output heart failure.
- Cardiomyopathy.
- Osteoporosis.

Map 5.1 Hyperthyroidism

What is hypothyroidism?

This occurs when there is too little circulating thyroid hormone in the body. There are many different causes of hypothyroidism.

Causes	
Type of hypothyroidism	**Cause**
Primary hypothyroidism	<ul><li>Iodine deficiency</li><li>Hashimoto's autoimmune thyroiditis</li><li>Post-thyroidectomy/radioactive iodine therapy</li><li>Drug induced, e.g. lithium, overtreatment of hyperthyroidism</li></ul>
Secondary hypothyroidism	<ul><li>Dysfunction of the hypothalamic–pituitary axis</li><li>Pituitary adenoma</li><li>Sheehan's syndrome (ischaemic necrosis of the pituitary gland after childbirth)</li><li>Infiltrative disease, e.g. tuberculosis and haemochromatosis</li></ul>

MAP 5.2 **Hypothyroidism**

Complications
- Hypercholesterolaemia.
- Complications in pregnancy, e.g. pre-eclampsia.
- Hyperthyroidism from overtreatment of hypothyroidism.
- Myxoedema coma.

Treatment
- Conservative: patient education.
- Medical: lifelong replacement of thyroid hormone with levothyroxine.

Investigations
- TFTs ($\uparrow$ TSH, $\downarrow$ T3 and $\downarrow$ T4).
- Thyroid antibodies.
- FBC (anaemia).
- U&Es.
- LFTs.
- Creatinine.
- Cholesterol.
- Guthrie test for congenital screening.

Signs and symptoms
- Weight gain.
- Cold skin/cold intolerance.
- Constipation.
- Dry skin.
- Thinning of hair.
- Bradycardia.
- Depression.
- Delayed reflexes.

Map 5.2 Hypothyroidism

What is thyroid carcinoma?

This is cancer that originates from follicular or parafollicular cells.

Causes

Malignant neoplasm. Increased risk with childhood neck irradiation.

Thyroid carcinomas may be classified histopathologically.

Histological appearance	% of thyroid cancer	Comment	
Papillary	70%	• Affects younger patients • Spreads to cervical lymph nodes	• Good prognosis
Follicular	20%	• More common in low iodine areas • Spreads to bone and lungs	• Good prognosis
Medullary	5%	• Arises from parafollicular cells • Calcitonin is a biochemical marker	• Associated with MEN syndrome • Spreads to lymph nodes
Anaplastic	<5%	• Affects older patients • Aggressive	• Spreads to lymph nodes • Poor prognosis
Other	-	• Lymphoma of the thyroid • Sarcoma of the thyroid	• Hürthle cell carcinoma (a variant of follicular carcinoma)

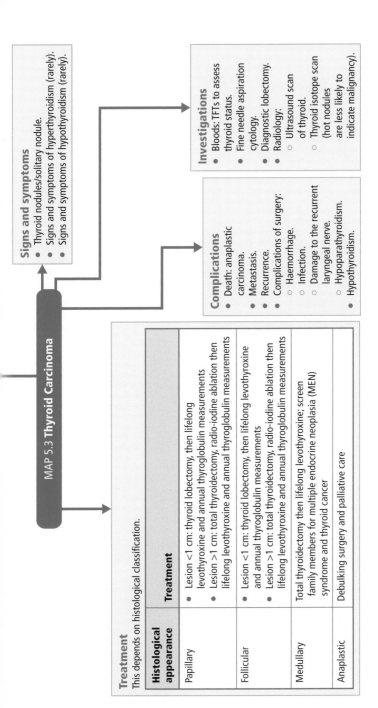

MAP 5.3 **Thyroid Carcinoma**

Signs and symptoms
- Thyroid nodules/solitary nodule.
- Signs and symptoms of hyperthyroidism (rarely).
- Signs and symptoms of hypothyroidism (rarely).

Investigations
- Bloods: TFTs to assess thyroid status.
- Fine needle aspiration cytology.
- Diagnostic lobectomy.
- Radiology:
  ○ Ultrasound scan of thyroid.
  ○ Thyroid isotope scan (hot nodules are less likely to indicate malignancy).

Complications
- Death: anaplastic carcinoma.
- Metastasis.
- Recurrence.
- Complications of surgery:
  ○ Haemorrhage.
  ○ Infection.
  ○ Damage to the recurrent laryngeal nerve.
  ○ Hypoparathyroidism.
- Hypothyroidism.

Treatment
This depends on histological classification.

Histological appearance	Treatment
Papillary	• Lesion <1 cm: thyroid lobectomy, then lifelong levothyroxine and annual thyroglobulin measurements • Lesion >1 cm: total thyroidectomy, radio-iodine ablation then lifelong levothyroxine and annual thyroglobulin measurements
Follicular	• Lesion <1 cm: thyroid lobectomy, then lifelong levothyroxine and annual thyroglobulin measurements • Lesion >1 cm: total thyroidectomy, radio-iodine ablation then lifelong levothyroxine and annual thyroglobulin measurements
Medullary	Total thyroidectomy then lifelong levothyroxine; screen family members for multiple endocrine neoplasia (MEN) syndrome and thyroid cancer
Anaplastic	Debulking surgery and palliative care

Map 5.4 Diabetes Mellitus (DM)

What is DM?

This is a metabolic condition in which the patient has hyperglycaemia due to insulin insensitivity or decreased insulin secretion.

- Type 1 DM: this is an autoimmune condition, which results in the destruction of the pancreatic beta cells resulting in no insulin production. This condition has a juvenile onset and is associated with HLA-DR3 and HLA-DR4. Patients are at risk of ketoacidosis.
- Type 2 DM: this occurs when patients gradually become insulin resistant or when the pancreatic beta cells fail to secrete enough insulin or both. It usually has a later life onset; however, the incidence is increasing in young populations due to environmental factors such as increasing obesity and sedentary lifestyle. Patients are at risk of developing a hyperosmolar state.
- Other cause of DM include: chronic pancreatitis, gestational DM and cystic fibrosis.

Treatment

Treatment	Type 1 DM	Type 2 DM
Conservative	Dietary advice BMI measurement Smoking cessation Decrease alcohol intake Regular blood glucose and HbA1c monitoring Encourage exercise	Dietary advice: high in complex carbohydrates, low in fat BMI measurement Smoking cessation Decrease alcohol intake Regular blood glucose and HbA1c monitoring Encourage exercise
Medical	See pages 80–82 for antidiabetic agents	See pages 80–82 for antidiabetic agents

MAP 5.4 **Diabetes Mellitus (DM)**

Investigations

Diagnostic investigations include:

- Fasting plasma glucose: >7 mmol/L (126 mg/dL).
- Random plasma glucose (plus DM symptoms): >11.1 mmol/L (200 mg/dL).
- HbA1c: >6.5% (48 mmol/mol).

Other tests include:

- Impaired glucose tolerance test (for borderline cases):
  - Fasting plasma glucose: <7 mmol/L (126 mg/dL) and at 2 h, after a 75 g oral glucose load, a level of 7.8–11 mmol/L (140–200 mg/dL).
  - Plasma glucose at 2 h: >11.1 mmol/L (>200 mg/dL).
- Impaired fasting glucose: plasma glucose: 5.6–6.9 mmol/L (110–126 mg/dL).

Signs and symptoms

- General: polyuria, polyphagia, polydipsia, blurred vision, glycosuria, signs of macrovascular and microvascular disease.
- More common in type 1 DM: acetone breath, weight loss, Kussmaul breathing, nausea and vomiting.

Complications

- Macrovascular: hypertension, increased risk of stroke, myocardial infarction, diabetic foot.
- Microvascular: nephropathy, peripheral neuropathy (glove and stocking distribution), retinopathy, erectile dysfunction.
- Psychological: depression.

TABLE 5.1 **Antidiabetic Agents**

For a full description of diabetes mellitus (DM) management and which drugs to use first line, please follow the website link provided for NICE guidelines in Appendix 2

Class of antidiabetic agent	Example	Mechanism of action	Uses	Side-effects	Contraindications	Drug interactions
Biguanides	Metformin	↑ Peripheral insulin sensitivity ↑ Glucose uptake into and use by skeletal muscle ↓ Hepatic gluconeogenesis ↓ Intestinal glucose absorption	Type 2 DM (first choice in overweight patients) Polycystic ovarian syndrome	Gastrointestinal tract (GIT) disturbance, e.g.diarrhoea Nausea Vomiting Lactic acidosis	Renal failure Cardiac failure Respiratory failure Hepatic failure (The above increase the risk of developing lactic acidosis)	Contrast agents Angiotensin converting enzyme (ACE) inhibitors Alcohol Nonsteroidal anti-inflammatory drugs (NSAIDs) Steroids
Sulphonylureas	Glipizide	Block potassium channels on the pancreatic beta cells, thus stimulating insulin release	Type 2 DM	GIT disturbance Hypoglycaemia Weight gain	Renal failure Hepatic failure Porphyria Pregnancy Breastfeeding	ACE inhibitors Alcohol NSAIDs Steroids
Meglitinides (glinides)	Repaglinide	Block potassium channels on the pancreatic beta cells, thus stimulating insulin release	Type 2 DM	Weight gain Hypoglycaemia	Hepatic failure Pregnancy Breastfeeding	Ciclosporin Trimethoprim Clarithromycin

Table 5.1 Antidiabetic Agents

Thiazolidinediones (glitazones)	Pioglitazone	Activates nuclear peroxisome proliferator-activated receptor (PPAR)	Type 2 DM	Weight gain Hypoglycaemia Hepatotoxicity Fracture risk	Type 1 DM Hepatic disease Heart failure Bladder cancer	Rifampicin Paclitaxel
Incretins	Exenatide	Analogue of glucagon-like peptide (GLP)-1	Type 2 DM	GIT disturbance, e.g. diarrhoea Acute pancreatitis	Thyroid cancer Multiple endocrine neoplasia (MEN) 2 syndrome	Bexarotene
	Saxagliptin	Inhibits dipeptidyl peptidase (DPP)-4	Type 2 DM	GIT disturbance, e.g. diarrhoea Infection of the respiratory and urinary tract Hepatotoxicity Peripheral oedema	History of serious hypersensitivity reaction	Thiazolidinedione
Alpha-glucosidase inhibitors	Acarbose	Inhibits alpha-glucosidase	Type 2 DM	GIT disturbance, e.g. diarrhoea	Inflammatory bowel disease (IBD) Intestinal obstruction Hepatic cirrhosis	Orlistat Pancreatin
Amylin analogues	Pramlintide	Analogue of amylin	Type 1 DM Type 2 DM	Severe hypoglycaemia	Gastroparesis Hypersensitivity to pramlintide	Acarbose

Continued overleaf

Table 5.1 Antidiabetic Agents

TABLE 5.1 **Antidiabetic Agents** (*Continued*)

Class of antidiabetic agent	Example	Mechanism of action	Uses	Side-effects	Contraindications	Drug interactions
Insulin therapy	Rapid acting, e.g. insulin lispro Short acting, e.g. soluble insulin Intermediate acting, e.g. isophane insulin Long acting, e.g. insulin glargine Biphasic, e.g. biphasic isophane insulin	Replaces insulin *Mechanism of action of insulin:* Insulin binds to tyrosine kinase receptors where it initiates 2 pathways by phosphorylation: 1 The MAP kinase signalling pathway: this is responsible for cell growth and proliferation. 2 The PI-3K signalling pathway: this is responsible for the transport of GLUT-4 receptors to the cell surface membrane; GLUT-4 transports glucose into the cell; this pathway is also responsible for protein, lipid and glycogen synthesis	Type 1 DM Type 2 DM	Weight gain Hypoglycaemia Localised lipoatrophy Hypokalaemia	Hypersensitivity to any of the therapy ingredients Hypoglycaemia	Repaglinide increases risk of myocardial infarction (MI) and hypoglycaemia Monoamine oxidase inhibitors may increase insulin secretion Corticosteroids decrease the effect of insulin Levothyroxine decreases the effect of insulin Thiazide diuretics decrease the effects of insulin

Table 5.1 Antidiabetic Agents

What is DI?

A disorder caused by low levels of or insensitivity to antidiuretic hormone (ADH) leading to polyuria. This can be cranial or nephrogenic in origin.

Causes

- Cranial: decreased ADH is released by the posterior pituitary gland. Remember this as **CIVIT**:
  - ○ **C**ongenital defect in ADH gene.
  - ○ **I**diopathic.
  - ○ **V**ascular.
  - ○ **I**nfection: meningoencephalitis.
  - ○ **T**umour (e.g. pituitary adenoma), **T**uberculosis and **T**rauma.
- Nephrogenic: the kidney does not respond to ADH. Remember this as **DIMC**:
  - ○ **D**rugs, e.g. lithium.
  - ○ **I**nherited.
  - ○ **M**etabolic ↓ potassium, ↑ calcium.
  - ○ **C**hronic renal disease.
  - (See also Figure 5.1.)

Signs and symptoms

- Polydipsia.
- Polyuria.
- Dehydration.

FIGURE 5.1 Causes of Diabetes Insipidus

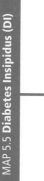

Posterior pituitary gland → ADH → Kidney → H_2O reabsorption

1 Cranial cause   2 Nephrogenic cause

MAP 5.5 **Diabetes Insipidus (DI)**

Continued overleaf

Map 5.5 Diabetes Insipidus (DI)

Map 5.5 Diabetes Insipidus (DI)

Complications

- Electrolyte imbalance.
- Dehydration.

MAP 5.5 **Diabetes Insipidus (DI)** (*Continued*)

Treatment

This depends on the cause:

- Conservative: patient education. Education on how to monitor fluid levels and dietary salt levels. Advise patients to wear a MedicAlert® bracelet.
- Medical:

Cranial cause	Nephrogenic cause
Desmopressin – a synthetic replacement for vasopressin; it increases the number of aquaporin-2 channels in the distal convoluted tubules and the collecting ducts. This increases water reabsorption	High-dose desmopressin
	Correction of electrolyte imbalances
	Thiazide diuretics
	Prostaglandin synthase inhibitors

- Surgical: excision of tumour if indicated.

Investigations

Investigation	Cranial cause	Nephrogenic cause
Plasma osmolality	↑	↑
Urine osmolality	↓	↓
Plasma Na⁺	↑	↑
24-h urine volume	>2 L	>2 L
Water deprivation test	Urine does not concentrate	Urine does not concentrate
After treatment with desmopressin	Urine becomes concentrated	Urine does not concentrate
MRI scan	Look for abnormality of the pituitary gland, e.g. tumour	

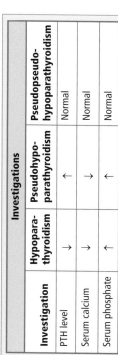

HYPOPARATHYROIDISM

What is it?

This occurs when too little PTH is produced from the parathyroid gland. It may be categorised into congenital, acquired, transient and inherited causes.

Causes	
Type	Cause
Congenital	DiGeorge syndrome (chromosome 22q11.2 deletion)
Acquired	Complication of parathyroidectomy or thyroidectomy
Transient	Neonates born prematurely
Inherited	Pseudohypoparathyroidism
	Pseudopseudohypoparathyroidism

Signs and symptoms

These depend on the cause: abdominal pain, myalgia, muscle spasm, seizures, fatigue, headaches, carpopedal spasm, Chvostek's sign, Trousseau's sign.

Treatment

- Conservative: diet high in calcium and low in phosphate. Support for parents.
- Medical: calcium and vitamin D supplements.

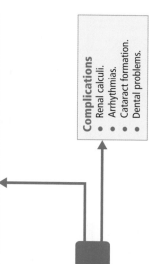

Investigations

	Investigations		
Investigation	Hypopara-thyroidism	Pseudohypo-parathyroidism	Pseudopseudo-hypoparathyroidism
PTH level	↓	↑	Normal
Serum calcium	↓	↓	Normal
Serum phosphate	↑	↑	Normal

Other investigations include:
- Bloods: FBC, U&Es, LFTs, creatinine, urea.
- ECG: arrhythmias.
- ECHO: cardiac structural defects (DiGeorge syndrome).
- Radiology: X-ray of hand (pseudohypoparathyroidism patients have shorter 4th and 5th metacarpals).

MAP 5.6
Hypoparathyroidism

Complications
- Renal calculi.
- Arrhythmias.
- Cataract formation.
- Dental problems.

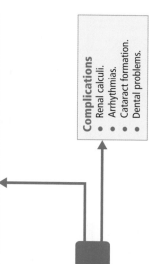

Map 5.6 Hypoparathyroidism

Map 5.7 Hyperparathyroidism

HYPERPARATHYROIDISM

What is it?

This occurs when too much parathyroid hormone (PTH) is produced from the parathyroid gland. It may be categorised into primary, secondary and tertiary causes.

Causes

Type	Cause
Primary	Parathyroid adenoma Parathyroid hyperplasia Parathyroid carcinoma Drug induced, e.g. lithium
Secondary	Vitamin D deficiency Chronic kidney injury
Tertiary	Prolonged secondary hyperparathyroidism

Signs and symptoms

These depend on the cause.

Primary – 'Bones, moans, groans and stones'	Secondary
Asymptomatic Bones, e.g. pain, osteoporosis Moans, e.g. depression, fatigue Groans, e.g. myalgia Stones, e.g. kidney stones	Osteomalacia Rickets Renal osteodystrophy

Investigations

Investigation	Primary	Secondary	Tertiary
PTH level	↑	↑	↑
Serum calcium	↑	↓	↑
Serum phosphate	↓	↑	↓

Other investigations include:
- Bloods: FBC, U&Es, LFTs, creatinine.
- Urine calcium level.
- Dual energy X-ray (DEXA) scan.
- Radiology:
  ○ Ultrasound scan of kidneys and neck.
  ○ Plain X-ray (for bone changes).
  ○ Parathyroid gland biopsy.

MAP 5.7
Hyperparathyroidism

Treatment

Type of treatment	Primary	Secondary	Tertiary
Conservative	Monitoring Increase oral fluid intake	Diet low in phosphate and high in calcium	–
Medical	Bisphosphonates	Calcimimetics, e.g. cinacalcet	–
Surgical	Parathyroidectomy	Parathyroidectomy if unresponsive to medical therapy	Para-thyroidectomy

Complications
- Renal calculi.
- Acute pancreatitis.
- Peptic ulceration.
- Calcification of the cornea.

Map 5.7 Hyperparathyroidism

Map 5.8 Cushing's Syndrome

What is Cushing's syndrome?

This is a collection of signs and symptoms that occur when a patient has long-term exposure to cortisol. There are many causes of Cushing's syndrome and they may be classified as exogenous or endogenous causes.

Type	Cause
Causes	
Exogenous	Iatrogenic, e.g. prescription of glucocorticoids for asthma
Endogenous	This may be split into adrenocorticotrophic hormone (ACTH) dependent and ACTH independent causes: • ACTH dependent: ○ Cushing's disease: this occurs when ACTH is produced from a pituitary adenoma. Use a low-dose dexamethasone test to confirm. ○ Ectopic ACTH production (usually from small cell lung cancer). • ACTH independent: **CARS:** ○ **C**ancer: adrenal adenoma. ○ **A**drenal nodular hyperplasia. ○ **R**are causes: McCune–Albright syndrome. ○ **S**teroid use.

MAP 5.8 Cushing's Syndrome

Signs and symptoms
- Moon face.
- Central obesity.
- Buffalo hump.
- Acne.
- Hypertension.
- Hyperglycaemia.
- Striae.
- Vertebral collapse.
- Proximal muscle wasting.
- Psychosis.

Investigations
- Diagnostic tests: urinary free cortisol, low-dose and high-dose dexamethasone suppression test.
- Bloods: FBC, U&Es, LFTs, glucose, lipid levels.
- Radiology: CXR (look for lung cancer and vertebral collapse).
- Other: dual energy X-ray (DEXA) scan.

Complications
- Osteoporosis.
- Diabetes mellitus.
- Hypertension.
- Immunosuppression.
- Cataracts.
- Striae formation.
- Ulcers.

Treatment
- Conservative: education about the condition. Advise patient to decrease alcohol consumption since alcohol increases cortisol levels.
- Medical: ketoconazole, metyrapone, mitotane. Treat complications such as hypertension and diabetes mellitus.
- Surgical: trans-sphenoidal surgery to remove pituitary adenoma or bilateral adrenalectomy to remove adrenal adenoma, if indicated.

FIGURE 5.2 **The Hypothalamic–Pituitary–Adrenal Axis**

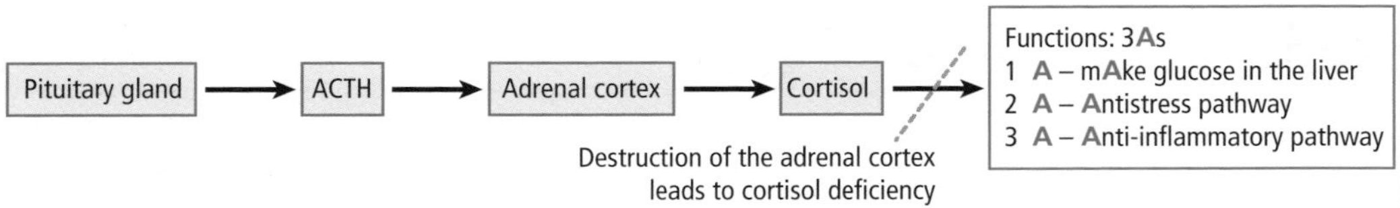

Pituitary gland → ACTH → Adrenal cortex → Cortisol

Destruction of the adrenal cortex
leads to cortisol deficiency

Functions: 3As
1 A – mAke glucose in the liver
2 A – Antistress pathway
3 A – Anti-inflammatory pathway

Map 5.9 Adrenal Insufficiency

What is adrenal insufficiency?

This occurs when the adrenal glands fail to produce sufficient steroid hormone. The causes of adrenal insufficiency may be categorised into primary and secondary adrenal failure.

Causes

Type	Cause
Primary	• Addison's disease; causes: **MAIL**: ○ **M**etastases from breast, lung and renal cancers. ○ **A**utoimmune. ○ **I**nfections, e.g. tuberculosis (commonest cause) and opportunistic infections, such as cytomegalovirus (CMV) in HIV patients. ○ **L**ymphomas. • Idiopathic. • Postadrenalectomy.
Secondary	• Prolonged prednisolone use. • Pituitary adenoma. • Sheehan's syndrome.

Signs and symptoms

- Unintentional weight loss.
- Myalgia.
- Weakness.
- Fatigue.
- Postural hypotension.
- Abdominal pain.
- Skin pigmentation.
- Body hair loss.
- Diarrhoea.
- Nausea.
- Vomiting.
- Depression.

Investigations

- Diagnostic tests:
  ○ Adrenocorticotrophic hormone (ACTH) and cortisol measurements.
  ○ Insulin tolerance test.
  ○ Short tetracosactide test aka Short Synacthen test.
- Bloods: FBC, U&Es ($\downarrow$ Na$^+$, $\uparrow$ K$^+$), LFTs, glucose, lipid levels, serum calcium.
- Radiology:
  ○ CXR (look for lung cancer).
  ○ CT and MRI scan of the adrenal glands.

Treatment

- Conservative: patient education. Patient must carry a steroid alert card.
- Medical: replace glucocorticoids, and mineralocorticoids with hydrocortisone and fludrocortisone; treat complications.
- Surgery: surgical excision of tumour, if indicated.

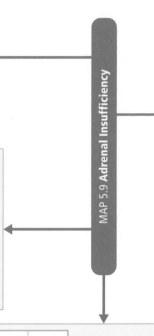

MAP 5.9 **Adrenal Insufficiency**

FIGURE 5.3 Anatomy of the Adrenal Cortex and Adrenal Medulla

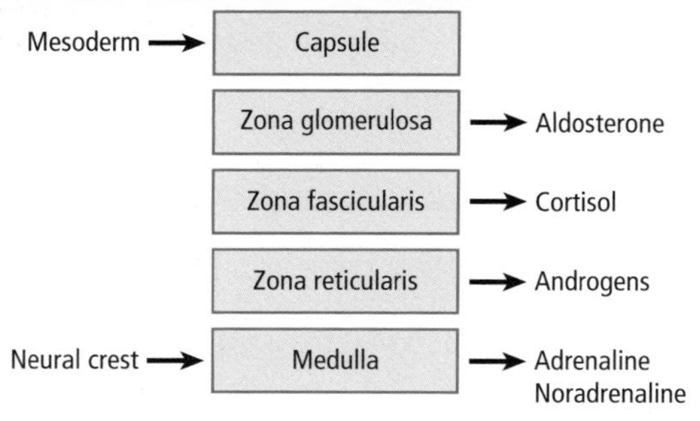

Mesoderm →

Capsule

Zona glomerulosa → Aldosterone

Zona fasciculceris → Cortisol

Zona reticularis → Androgens

Neural crest →

Medulla → Adrenaline / Noradrenaline

Complications

- Adrenal crisis.
- Hyperkalaemia.
- Hypoglycaemia.
- Eosinophilia.
- Alopecia.
- Addison's disease is associated with other conditions such as

3PGH:

- ○ **P**ernicious anaemia.
- ○ **P**rimary ovarian failure.
- ○ **P**olyglandular syndrome.
- ○ **G**raves' disease.
- ○ **H**ashimoto's thyroiditis.

Map 5.9 Adrenal Insufficiency

The Endocrine System

Map 5.10 Acromegaly

What is acromegaly?

Acromegaly is a syndrome that results from excessive growth hormone (GH) production after fusion of the epiphyseal plates. Excess GH produced before epiphyseal plate fusion causes gigantism.

Causes

- Pituitary adenoma (most common).
- GH releasing hormone (GHRH) production from bronchial carcinoid.

Signs and symptoms

- Increased jaw size.
- Increased hand size.
- Macroglossia.
- Lower pitch of voice.
- Carpal tunnel syndrome.
- Ask to see old photographs of the patient and note changes in appearance.

Investigations

- Bloods: FBC, U&Es, creatinine, LFTs, glucose, lipid levels, GH levels, glucose tolerance test, insulin-like growth factor (IGF)-1 levels(raised), prolactin levels.
- Radiology:
  ○ CXR.
  ○ CT and MRI scan.
- ECG and ECHO: assess for cardiac complications, e.g. cardiomyopathy.
- Visual field testing: bilateral hemianopia.

MAP 5.10 **Acromegaly**

Complications

- Increased risk of cardiovascular disease.
- Hypertension.
- Diabetes mellitus.
- Increased risk of colon cancer.
- Erectile dysfunction.
- Postsurgical, e.g. infection, cerebrospinal fluid (CSF) leak.

Treatment

- Conservative: patient education. Inform the patient that bone changes will not revert after treatment.
- Medical:
  ○ Somatostatin analogues, e.g. octreotide.
  ○ Dopamine agonists, e.g. cabergoline.
  ○ GH receptor antagonists, e.g. pegvisomant.
- Surgery: trans-sphenoidal surgical excision of the adenoma is the treatment of choice.

Map 6.1 Anaemia

MAP 6.1 Anaemia

What is anaemia?

Anaemia occurs when the haemoglobin (Hb) concentration is low.
This condition may be classified as microcytic, macrocytic or normocytic.

TABLE 6.1 Anaemia

Type of anaemia	Causes	Symptoms	Signs	Investigations	Treatment	Complications
Microcytic	Iron deficiency of varying cause, e.g. • Menorrhagia • Pregnancy • Gastrointestinal tract malignancy • Oesophagitis • Gastro-oesophageal reflux disease • Coeliac disease • Hookworm • Schistosomiasis • Diet low in iron Thalassaemia: see page 96	Fatigue Palpitations Headache Dyspnoea	Pallor Nail changes, e.g. koilonychia Angular cheilitis Atrophic glossitis	FBC • Microcytic, hypochromic anaemia • ↓ MCV (<80 fL) • ↓ MCH • ↓ Ferritin • ↓ Iron • ↑ Total iron binding capacity (TIBC) Blood film: anisocytosis and poikilocytosis Investigate causes, e.g. endoscopy, stool microscopy, barium enema	Treat cause Ferrous sulphate	Fatigue Increased risk of infection Heart failure
Macrocytic	Remember these as **FAT RBC:** **F**olate deficiency **A**lcohol **T**hyroid (hypothyroidism)	Fatigue Palpitations Headache Dyspnoea Irritability Depression	Pallor Glossitis Angular cheilitis Paraesthesiae Subacute degeneration of the spinal cord	FBC • ↓ Hb • ↑ MCV (>96 fL) • ↓ Vitamin B$_{12}$ • ↓ Folate • ↑ Reticulocytes • ↓ Platelets (if severe)	Treat cause If pernicious anaemia then treat with hydroxocobalamin injections	Fatigue Heart failure Splenomegaly Neuropsychiatric and neurological complications

	Causes	Symptoms	Signs	Investigations	Treatment	Complications
	Reticulocytosis **B**$_{12}$ (vitamin B$_{12}$ deficiency)/ pernicious anaemia **C**ytotoxic drugs			• ↓ WCC (if severe) Blood film: hypersegmented polymorphs (folate and vitamin B$_{12}$ deficiency); target cells observed in liver disease		Fatigue Heart failure
Normocytic	Haemolytic anaemia of varying cause, e.g. • Glucose-6-phosphate dehydrogenase deficiency • Hereditary spherocytosis • Erythroblastosis fetalis • Sickle cell disease • Warm antibody autoimmune haemolytic anaemia and cold agglutinin disease • Anaemia of chronic disease, e.g. rheumatoid arthritis Aplastic anaemia	Fatigue Palpitations Headache Dyspnoea Symptoms of underlying disease	Pallor Signs of underlying disease	FBC • ↓ Hb • Normal MCV • Normal or ↑ ferritin	Treat cause	

Table 6.1 Anaemia

MAP 6.2 Thalassaemia

Map 6.2 Thalassaemia

What is thalassaemia?

Thalassaemias are genetic conditions, inherited in an autosomal recessive pattern, that produce a picture of microcytic anaemia due to a problem in globin chain production. This subsequently alters haemoglobin (Hb) synthesis. Thalassaemia may be classified into α-thalassaemia and β-thalassaemia.

TABLE 6.2 Thalassaemia

Types of thalassaemia	Populations affected	Causes	Investigations	Treatment	Complications
α-thalassaemia	More prominent in African and Asian populations	↓ α-globin synthesis due to α-globin gene mutation on chromosome 16; this subsequently results in excess β-globin production In α-thalassaemia any number between 1 and 4 genes may be deleted: • 1 gene deleted = no significant anaemia • 2 genes deleted = trait disease • 3 genes deleted = HbH disease	Blood films: in α-thalassaemia target cells (or Mexican hat cells) may be seen FBC: • Microcytic, hypochromic anaemia • ↓ MCV • ↓ MCH • Ferritin normal • Iron normal Hb electrophoresis: ↑ HbA_2 and ↑ HbF High performance liquid chromatography Radiology: X-ray for bone abnormalities, e.g. frontal bossing	Conservative: patient education, genetic counselling Medical: • Management of α-thalassaemia and β-thalassaemia is based on patient symptoms and overall state of health • Transfusions are usually required when Hb <7 g/dL or when the patient is highly symptomatic	Iron overload Splenomegaly Increased risk of infection Heart failure Arrhythmias Bone abnormalities, e.g. cranial bossing Gallstones

β-thalassaemia	More prominent in European populations	Point mutatioin in β-globin chain on chromosome 11; this subsequently results in excess α-globin production	
		β-thalassaemia may be subdivided into 3 different traits:	
		1 Minor: usually asymptomatic; carrier state; mild anaemia	
		2 Intermediate: moderate anaemia; no blood transfusions required	
		3 Major: aka Cooley's anaemia; abnormalities in all β-globin chains results in severe anaemia; characteristic cranial bossing seen due to extramedullary haematopoiesis	

- 4 genes deleted = death – Bart's hydrops fetalis

- Patients who have repeated blood transfusions are at risk of haemochromatosis and, therefore, require iron chelation therapy, e.g. desferroxamine.

Surgical:
- Splenectomy
- Stem cell transplant

Table 6.2 Thalassaemia

Map 6.3 Bleeding Disorders

HAEMOPHILIA

What is haemophilia?

This is an inherited condition that impairs the body's ability to coagulate the blood.

Causes

This is a hereditary condition. There are two forms of haemophilia:

- Type A: lack of factor VIII.
- Type B: lack of factor IX.

Investigations

- Normal prothrombin time, ↑ partial thromboplastin time.

Treatment

- Conservative: patient education. Avoid aspirin, NSAIDs, heparin and warfarin.
- Medical: replace deficient clotting factor with regular infusions.

CLOT FORMATION

This consists of 4 steps. Defects in steps 2–4 may lead to a bleeding disorder.

1. Vessel constriction.
2. Platelet adhesion and aggregation: Glanzmann's thrombasthenia, von Willebrand disease, Bernard–Soulier syndrome.
3. Blood coagulation: haemophilia.
4. Fibrinolysis: antiplasmin deficiency.

BERNARD–SOULIER SYNDROME

What is Bernard–Soulier syndrome?

This is an autosomal recessive bleeding disorder.

Causes

This is a hereditary condition that leads to deficiency of glycoprotein (Gp) Ib.

Investigations

- ↑ Bleeding time, normal or ↓ platelet count.

Treatment

- Conservative: patient education.
- Medical:
  - Desmopressin may decrease bleeding time.
  - Recombinant activated factor VII.

MAP 6.3 **Bleeding Disorders**

VITAMIN K INSUFFICIENCY
What is vitamin K insufficiency?
This avitaminosis occurs when there is decreased vitamin K₁ or vitamin K₂ or both. This results in:

- ↓ Synthesis of factors II, VII, IX and X.
- ↓ Synthesis of proteins C and S.

Causes
- Drugs, e.g. warfarin.
- Malnutrition.
- Malabsorption.
- Alcoholism.
- Cystic fibrosis.
- Chronic kidney injury.
- Cholestatic disease.

Investigations
- ↑ Prothrombin time, normal or ↑ partial thromboplastin time.

Treatment
- Conservative – patient education. Dietary advice about food rich in vitamin K
- Medical – treat cause. Vitamin K supplements.

GLANZMANN'S THROMBASTHENIA
What is Glanzmann's thrombasthenia?
This is a rare autosomal recessive or acquired autoimmune condition in which platelets are deficient of GpIIb/IIIa. GpIIb/IIIa binds fibrinogen.

Causes
Disease of hereditary or acquired autoimmune cause.

Investigations
- ↑ Bleeding time.

Treatment
- Conservative: patient education. Avoid aspirin and nonsteroidal anti-inflammatory drugs (NSAIDs).
- Medical:
  - Desmopressin.
  - Recombinant activated factor VII.

VON WILLEBRAND DISEASE
What is von Willebrand disease?
This is the most common hereditary coagulation disorder, which involves a defect in von Willebrand factor (VWF). The function of von Willebrand factor is to bind GpIb receptor on platelets to subendothelial collagen.

Causes
Hereditary condition. There are many different types of von Willebrand disease, but the most common are type 1, type 2, type 3 and type Normandy.

Investigations
- ↑ Activated partial thromboplastin time,
- ↑ Bleeding time, normal prothrombin time,
- ↓ VWF antigen, ↓ factor VIIIc.

Treatment
- Conservative: patient education. Avoid aspirin and NSAIDs.
- Medical: desmopressin may be useful, but is not helpful in type 3 von Willebrand disease.

Map 6.3 Bleeding Disorders

Map 6.4 Leukaemia

What is leukaemia?

This is a rare neoplasm of the blood or bone marrow. It is classified into lymphoid and myeloid neoplasms that may present chronically or acutely. These 4 classifications are:

1 Acute lymphoblastic leukaemia (ALL).
2 Chronic lymphocytic leukaemia (CLL).
3 Acute myeloid leukaemia (AML).
4 Chronic myeloid leukaemia (CML).

Causes

Neoplasm	Cause	Comment
ALL	Possibly a genetic susceptibility coupled with an environmental trigger	Commonest cancer in children Often spreads to central nervous system Associations – **DIP:** • **D**own's syndrome • **I**onising radiation • **P**regnancy
CLL	Exact cause unknown	Usually affects adults over 60 years old Affects B lymphocytes Positive ZAP-70 marker is associated with a worse prognosis
AML	Exact cause unknown Risk factors include: • Myeloproliferative disease • Alkylating agents • Ionising radiation exposure • Down's syndrome	Commonest leukaemia in adults Rapidly progressing Auer rods on microscopy are diagnostic
CML	Exact cause unknown Risk factor: ionising radiation exposure	Usually affects males 40–60 years old 80% associated with the Philadelphia chromosome t[9;22], forming *bcr-abl* fusion gene

Signs and symptoms

Neoplasm	Clinical features
ALL	Bone marrow failure Bruising Shortness of breath Purpura Malaise Weight loss Night sweats
CLL	Asymptomatic Bone marrow failure Nontender lymphadenopathy Hepatosplenomegaly Malaise Weight loss Night sweats

MAP 6.4 Leukaemia

Complications
- Death.
- Increased risk of infection.
- Haemorrhage: pulmonary, intracranial.
- Depression.
- Complication of chemotherapy.

Investigations
- Bloods: FBC, WCC, platelets, U&Es, LFTs, ESR, CRP.
- Bone marrow biopsy, lymph node biopsy.
- Radiology: X-ray, ultrasound scan, CT scan, MRI.
- AML and ALL are classified using the French–American–British (FAB) classification.

AML	Bone marrow failure	
	Malaise	
	Weight loss	
	Night sweats	
CML	Bone marrow failure	
	Hepatosplenomegaly	
	Malaise	
	Weight loss	
	Night sweats	

Treatment

Treatment	ALL	CLL	AML	CML
Conservative	Patient education; refer to Macmillan nurses			
Medical	Induce remission and maintenance To induce remission: • Dexamethasone • Vincristine • Anthracycline antibiotics • Cyclophosphamide Maintenance: • Methotrexate • Mercaptopurine • Cytarabine • Hydrocortisone	Chlorambucil Fludarabine Rituximab Prednisolone Cyclophosphamide	Patients <60 years: chemotherapy with an anthracycline and cytarabine or methotrexate Patients >60 years: palliative anthracycline, cytarabine or mitoxantrone If M3 type AML, i.e. acute promyelocytic leukaemia (APML), then add all-trans retinoic acid to the therapeutic regime	Imatinib Patients <60 years may be considered for allogeneic stem cell transplantation Other treatments include alpha-interferon, vincristine, prednisolone, cytarabine and daunorubicin

Map 6.4 Leukaemia

102 **Haematology**

Map 6.5 Hodgkin's vs. Non-Hodgkin's Lymphoma

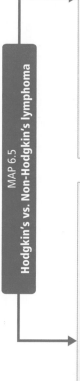

MAP 6.5
Hodgkin's vs. Non-Hodgkin's Lymphoma

HODGKIN'S LYMPHOMA
What is hodgkin's lymphoma?
This is a group of uncommon malignancies; the 4 most common histological subtypes are:

1 Lymphocyte-predominant.
2 Nodular sclerosing.
3 Mixed cellularity.
4 Lymphocyte-depleted.

Cause
Exact cause is unknown.
Risk factors include:
- Male sex.
- Infection with Epstein–Barr virus (EBV).
- Immunosuppression, e.g. HIV patients.
- Exotoxin exposure.

Signs and symptoms
- Painless lymphadenopathy.
- Unintentional weight loss.
- Fever (constitutional '**B** signs': fever >38°C, night sweats, weight loss).

NON-HODGKIN'S LYMPHOMA
What is non-Hodgkin's lymphoma?
This is a group of malignancies that are either B cell or T cell in origin.

B cell neoplasms	T cell neoplasms
Burkitt's lymphoma: • Associated with EBV • t[8;14] Diffuse large B cell lymphoma Mantle cell lymphoma: t[11;14] Follicular lymphoma: • t[14;18] • bcl-2 expression	Adult T cell lymphoma; caused by human T-lymphotrophic virus-1 (HTLV-1) Sézary syndrome

Cause
Exact cause is unknown.
Risk factors include:
- Male sex.
- Infection, e.g. EBV, *Helicobacter pylori*, human herpes virus (HHV)-8, hepatitis C.
- Immunosuppression, e.g. HIV patients.

- Dyspnoea.
- Splenomegaly.
- Hepatomegaly.

Investigations

- Bloods: FBC, WCC, U&Es, CRP, ESR, lactate dehydrogenase, creatinine, alkaline phosphatase, serum cytokine levels.
- Histology: Reed–Sternberg cells are seen.
- Radiology: X-ray, CT scan, PET scan.
- Other: lymph node biopsy (Ann Arbor classification).

Treatment

- Conservative: patient education and referral to Macmillan nurses.
- Medical: depends on Ann Arbor classification; AVBD regimen: doxorubicin, vinblastine, bleomycin, dacarbazine; BEACOPP regimen: bleomycin, etoposide, doxorubicin, cyclophosphamide, vincristine, procarbazine, prednisolone.

Complications

- Increased risk of infection.
- Recurrence and metastasis.
- Increased risk of cardiovascular disease.
- Complications of chemotherapy.
- Neurological complications.

Signs and symptoms

- Painless lymphadenopathy.
- Unintentional weight loss.
- Fever.
- Dyspnoea.
- Splenomegaly.
- Hepatomegaly.

Investigations

- Bloods: FBC, WCC, U&Es, CRP, ESR, lactate dehydrogenase, creatinine, alkaline phosphatase, serum cytokine levels, soluble CD25 level.
- Radiology: X-ray, CT scan, PET scan.
- Other: lymph node biopsy (Ann Arbor classification).

Treatment

- Conservative: patient education and referral to Macmillan nurses.
- Medical: depends on causes and severity (Ann Arbor classification); R-CHOP regimen: rituximab, cyclophosphamide, hydroxydaunomycin, vincristine, prednisolone; other agents used are cisplatin, etoposide and methotrexate.

Complications

- Increased risk of infection.
- Recurrence and metastasis.
- Increased risk of cardiovascular disease.
- Complications of chemotherapy.
- Neurological complications.

Map 6.5 Hodgkin's vs. Non-Hodgkin's Lymphoma

Map 6.6 Myeloma

What is myeloma?
This is a malignant neoplasm of the plasma cells.

Causes
Exact cause is unknown. Risk factors include:
- Monoclonal gammopathy of unknown significance.
- Pernicious anaemia.
- History of thyroid cancer.
- Exposure to certain exotoxins, e.g. benzene, Agent Orange.
- Past history of radiation exposure.

Signs and symptoms
- Fatigue.
- Unintentional weight loss.
- Pathological fractures.
- Vertebral collapse (may lead to spinal cord compression).
- Hypercalcaemia.
- Anaemia.
- Infection.
- Renal impairment.
- Bruising.

Investigations
- Bloods: FBC (normocytic, normochromic anaemia), U&Es, creatinine, LFTs, ESR, CRP, calcium levels, alkaline phosphatase, beta-2 microglobulin.
- Blood film: rouleaux formation.
- Serum and urine electrophoresis: paraprotein (M protein), Bence Jones proteinuria.
- Bone marrow biopsy.
- Radiology:
  ○ X-ray for bone deformities, e.g. pepper pot skull and generalised skeletal osteopaenia.
  ○ MRI scan may be useful.

MAP 6.6 Myeloma

Complications
- Spinal cord compression.
- Pathological fracture.
- Hypercalcaemia.
- Acute kidney injury.
- Increased risk of infection.
- Anaemia.

Treatment
- Conservative: patient education. Refer to Macmillan nurses.
- Medical: medical therapy in multiple myeloma depends on the age of the patient and their state of health. If they are <70 years and without significant co-morbidities then they are eligible for autologous bone marrow transplant, which is the most effective treatment. This involves an induction phase using the VAD regimen: vincristine, adriamycin, dexamethasone. After transplant the patient receives long-term therapy with melphalan.
  ○ Patients who are ineligible for autologous bone marrow transplant receive long-term treatment with melphalan and prednisolone.
  ○ Other medical therapy is targeted to treating symptoms: analgesia, bisphosphonates, prednisolone, blood transfusion.
  ○ Radiotherapy may be required to treat bone pain and spinal cord compression.
- Surgical: kyphoplasty may be required.

Infectious Disease

What is malaria?

This is an infectious disease caused by parasitic *Plasmodium*, which is spread by the female *Anopheles* mosquito.

Causes

- *Plasmodium falciparum*: most severe form.
  Causes cerebral malaria.
- *P. ovale*: may lie dormant within the liver as hypnozoites.
- *P. vivax*: may lie dormant within the liver as hypnozoites.
- *P. malariae*.
- *P. knowlesi*: very rare.

Signs and symptoms

- Fatigue.
- Night sweats.
- Flu-like symptoms.
- Diarrhoea.
- Nausea.
- Vomiting.
- Anaemia.
- Splenomegaly.
- Seizures (cerebral malaria or secondary to fever).

Treatment

- Conservative; patient education. Prevention of disease, e.g. mosquito nets and repellent sprays.
- Medical: prophylactic and therapeutic.
  Treatment is dependent on *Plasmodium* species:
  1 Inhibit haem polymerase:
     ○ Chloroquine.
     ○ Quinine.
  2 Blood schizonticide:
     ○ Mefloquine (Lariam).
     ○ Primaquine.
     ○ Malarone.
  3 Inhibits plasmodial protein synthesis: doxycycline.
  4 Inhibits dihydrofolate reductase: pyrimethamine.
  5 Inhibits falciparum sarcoplasmic–endoplasmic reticulum calcium ATPase: artemether (always used with lumefantrine).
  6 Inhibits haem metabolism: lumefantrine.
- Surgical: splenectomy, if indicated.

Investigations

- Bloods: FBC, U&Es, creatinine, LFTs, ESR, CRP.
- Blood film.
- Real-time PCR.
- Antigen detection kits.

Complications

- Cerebral malaria.
- Anaemia.
- Hepatic failure.
- Splenomegaly.
- Shock.
- Acute kidney injury.
- Dehydration.
- Acute respiratory distress syndrome (ARDS).

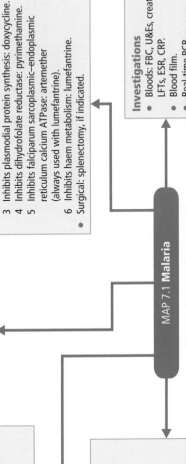

MAP 7.1 Malaria

Map 7.1 Malaria

FIGURE 7.1 Malaria Lifecycle

Infected mosquito bites human host

Sporozoites enter the circulatory system

The sporozoites travel in the blood to the liver where they infect hepatocytes

Within the hepatocyte the sporozoites mature into schizonts, which produce many merozoites. *P. vivax* has an additional dormant stage where the sporozoites become hypnozoites.

These merozoites replicate until their vast numbers eventually rupture the hepatocytes. In doing this the merozoites enter the bloodstream and infect red blood cells

Malaria lifecycle: transmitted by female *Anopheles* mosquito

Within the red blood cells merozoites continue to replicate until the red blood cells rupture

Some of these red blood cells become gametocytes, which remain in the blood for a few days. During this time the gametocytes may be transferred to a mosquito that feeds on this infected human

Within the mosquito the gametocytes turn into sporozoites and the mosquito is now a vector of disease

Figure 7.1 Malaria Lifecycle

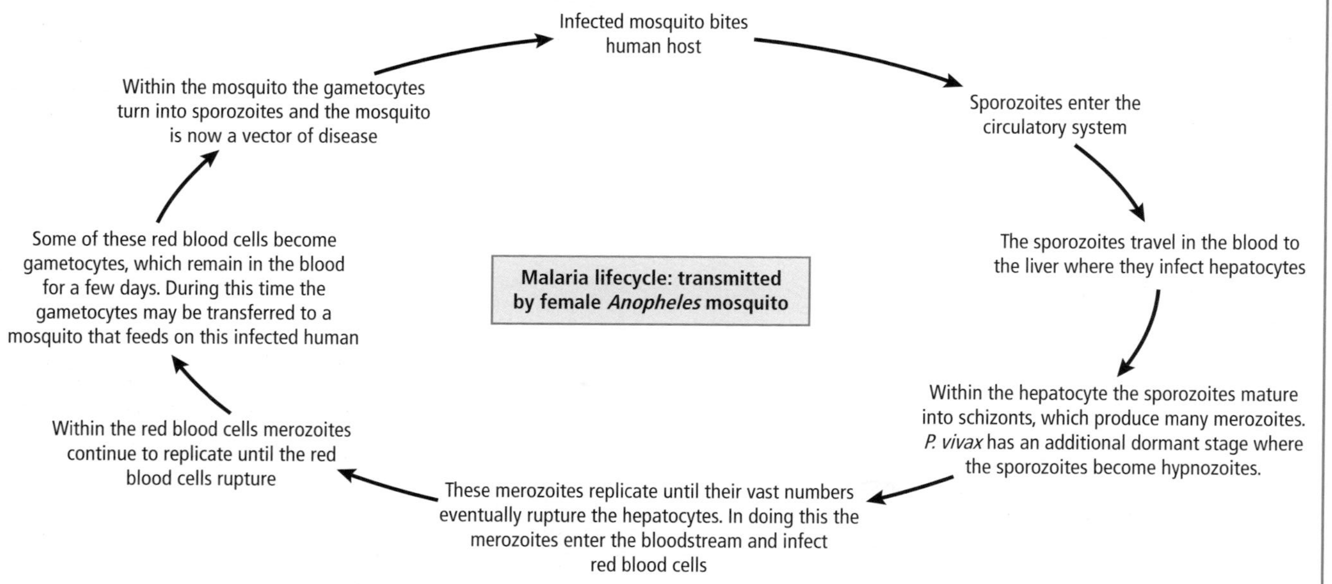

Map 7.2 Tuberculosis (TB)

What is TB?

TB is a granulomatous disease that may affect any organ, but most commonly affects the lungs since it is transmitted via aerosol droplets.

Causes

Mycobacterium tuberculosis (acid-fast bacillus).

Pathophysiology

- Primary pulmonary TB:
  ○ Initial TB infection.
  ○ Ghon focus formation in upper lobes.
  ○ Hilar lymphadenopathy.
- Secondary pulmonary TB:
  ○ Occurs after primary infection.
  ○ Dormant TB is reactivated.
  ○ Fibrocaseous lesions.
- Other forms of TB:
  ○ Miliary.
  ○ Genitourinary.
  ○ Bone, e.g. Pott's disease of the spine.
  ○ Peritoneal.
  ○ Meningitis.

Investigations

- Sputum culture:
  ○ Ogawa/Löwenstein–Jensen medium.
- Sputum stain: Ziehl–Neelsen stain.
- Transbronchial biopsy: granulomas are diagnostic.
- Pleural fluid analysis and biopsy.
- Radiology: X-ray for infiltrates and cavitations. Lesions described as millet seeds in miliary TB.

Treatment

- Conservative: patient education, especially the importance of complying with medical therapy.
- Medical – remember **RIPE**:
  ○ **R**ifampicin.
  ○ **I**soniazid.
  ○ **P**yrazinamide.
  ○ **E**thambutol.

Other drugs that may be used in therapy include: streptomycin, quinolones, amikacin and capreomycin.

- Surgical: depends on location, e.g. for pulmonary TB consider lobectomy.

Signs and symptoms

- Cough.
- Haemoptysis.
- Weight loss.
- Night sweats.
- Fever.

Complications

- Dissemination to other organs.
- Death.

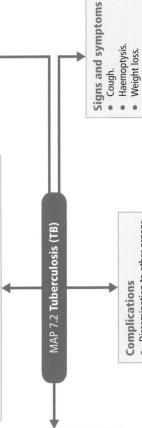

MAP 7.2 Tuberculosis (TB)

FIGURE 7.2 **Mode of Infection of Pulmonary TB**

Mode of infection

Droplets inhaled

↓

Bacteria colonise alveoli

↓

Bacteria engulfed by macrophages

↓

Multiplication of bacteria within macrophages

↓

Granulomas form around *M. tuberculosis* (caseous necrosis)

Immunocompetent patients – caseous necrosis produces conditions that decrease the growth of bacteria, e.g. lowered oxygen and pH levels

↓

Latency

Nonimmunocompetent patients – granuloma formation does not contain bacteria

↓

Liquefaction of necrotic tissue

↓

Coughing of infectious droplets since the liquified necrotic tissue drains into the bronchus

Figure 7.2 Mode of Infection of Pulmonary TB

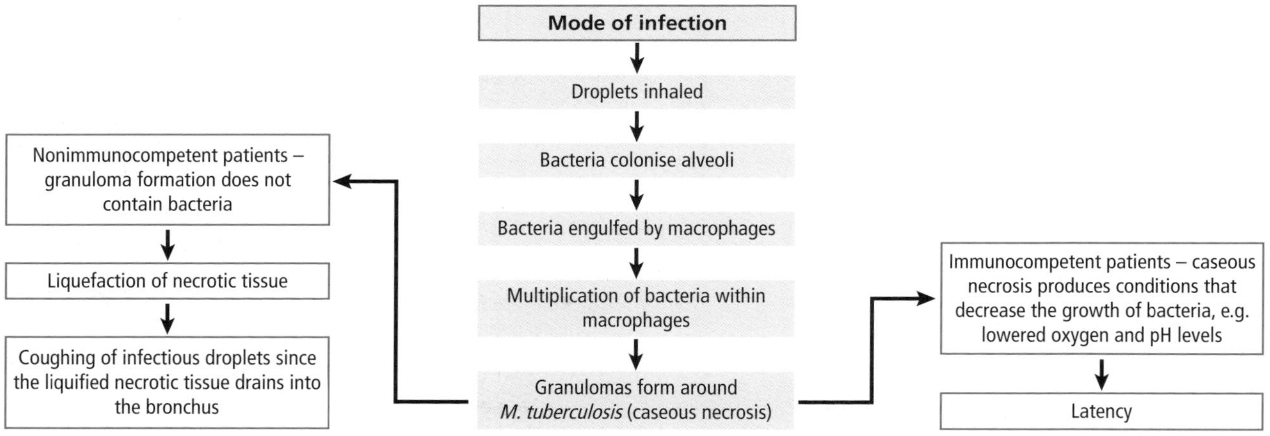

Map 7.3 Human Herpes Virus (HHV)

Note
HHV-1 and HHV-2 may affect both the mouth and the genitals.

HHV-2
- Herpes genitalis.

HHV-1
- Herpes labialis.

Investigations
A clinical diagnosis, which may be confirmed by culturing the virus and by immunofluorescence.

Treatment
- Conservative: patient education and methods to reduce spread.
- Medical: antiviral medications, e.g. aciclovir and famciclovir.

MAP 7.3 **Human Herpes Virus (HHV)**

HHV-8
- Kaposi's sarcoma (associated with HIV).

HHV-7
- Belongs to the subfamily betaherpesviridae.
- It is closely related to HHV-6.

HHV-6
- Roseola infantum.

Cytomegalovirus (HHV-5)
- Mononucleosis (negative Monospot test).
- Typically seen in immunocompromised patients.
- Transmitted via sexual contact, saliva, urine, transplant, transfusion and congenitally.

Epstein–Barr virus (HHV-4)
- Infectious mononucleosis–'kissing disease' (positive Monospot test).
- Associated with Burkitt's lymphoma.
- Associated with nasopharyngeal carcinoma.
- Transmitted via droplet infection and saliva.

Varicella zoster virus (HHV-3)
- Chickenpox.
- Shingles.

Map 7.3 Human Herpes Virus (HHV)

Map 7.4 Human Immunodeficiency Virus (HIV)

Complications

- Increased risk of opportunistic infections:
  - Toxoplasmosis.
  - CMV, e.g. retinitis.
  - *Pneumocystis jiroveci* pneumonia.
  - Cryptococcal meningitis.
  - *Mycobacterium avium* complex.
  - *Candida*.
  - Aspergillosis.
- Increased risk of malignancies:
  - Kaposi's sarcoma.
  - Non-Hodgkin's lymphoma.
  - Cervical cancer.
  - Anal cancer.

Investigations

- Bloods: FBC, U&Es, LFTs, lipids, glucose, HLA-B*5701 status, lymphocyte subsets.
- HIV specific:
  - Enzyme-linked immunosorbent assay (ELISA).
  - Western blot test.
  - Immunofluorescence assay (IFA).
  - Nucleic acid testing.
- Virology screen: HIV antibody, HIV viral load, HIV genotype, hepatitis serology, cytomegalovirus (CMV) antibody, syphilis screen.
- Other infection, e.g. tuberculosis if indicated.

What is HIV?

HIV is an RNA retrovirus of the lentivirus genus. This virus causes acquired immunodeficiency syndrome (AIDS).

Causes

There are two types of HIV:

1 HIV-1:
- Type M: A–J prevalent in Europe, America, Australia and sub-Saharan Africa.
- Type O: mainly in Cameroon.
2 HIV-2: predominantly confined to West Africa.

Transmission

- Unprotected sexual intercourse.
- Shared contaminated needles.
- Contaminated blood transfusions.
- Vertical transmission from mother to child.
The virus crosses the placenta and is transmitted through breast milk.

MAP 7.4 **Human Immunodeficiency Virus (HIV)**

Treatment

- Conservative: patient education including transmission reduction advice. Contact tracing. Psychological support.
- Medical: highly active antiretroviral therapy (HAART): either 2 × NRTIs combined with 1 × NNRTI or 2 × NRTIs combined with 1 × PIs or 1 × II:
  - Nucleoside reverse transcriptase inhibitor (NRTI), e.g. zidovudine.
  - Non-nucleoside reverse transcriptase inhibitor (NNRTI), e.g. nevirapine.
  - Protease inhibitor (PI), e.g. indinavir.
  - Integrase inhibitor (II), e.g. raltegravir.

Infection process

- gp120 antigen on HIV binds to CD4+ receptors on the T cell.
- This process produces a conformational change and the need to bind to a co-receptor: CCR5 or CXCR4.
- gp41 binds to the co-receptor.
- This binding causes 'six-helix bundle formation' and fusion of the viral and host membranes.
- Disintegration of the viral capsid occurs causing viral RNA to be released into the human cell.
- Double-stranded RNA is produced and this process is catalysed by viral reverse transcriptase.
- Double-stranded RNA is integrated into host DNA using integrase enzyme.
- Host cell now manufactures new virions by long terminal repeat sequences and genes *tat* and *rev*.

Genes required for viral replication
Remember **PEG**

- **p**ol: encodes reverse transcriptase and integrase.
- **e**nv: encodes envelope proteins, e.g. gp120.
- **g**ag: encodes viral structural proteins.

Map 7.4 Human Immunodeficiency Virus (HIV)

Map 7.5 Sexually Transmitted Infections (STIs)

TRICHOMONAS VAGINALIS
What is *Trichomonas vaginalis*?
It is an anaerobic protozoon, which causes trichomoniasis. Symptoms include a fishy bubbly thin discharge and on speculum examination 'strawberry' cervix is visible.

Investigations
● Cervical smear.
● Rapid antigen testing.
● PCR technique.

Treatment
Metronidazole. Intravaginal clotrimazole during pregnancy.

Complications
● Increased risk of HIV infection
● Increased risk of cervical cancer.
● Increased risk of preterm delivery.

GARDNERELLA VAGINALIS
What is *Gardnerella vaginalis*?
This is a facultative anaerobic coccobacillus that causes bacterial vaginosis ('fishy odour' and grey discharge). N.B. This is NOT an STI but does cause vaginal discharge and, as such, is included in differential diagnosis with chlamydia and gonorrhoea.

Investigations
● Microscopy – clue cells observed.

Treatment
● Metronidazole or clindamycin.

Complications
● Rarely causes complications.

TREPONEMA PALLIDUM
What is *Treponema pallidum*?
This is a spirochaete that causes syphilis.
Infection occurs in 3 stages:
1 Chancre: painless superficial ulceration.
2 Disseminated disease: systemic involvement, rash seen on palms and soles.
3 Cardiac and neurological involvement.

Investigations
● Venereal Disease Research Laboratory (VDRL) test.
● Rapid plasma reagin (RPR) test.
● *Treponema pallidum* particle agglutination.
● Fluorescent treponemal antibody absorption (FTA) test.
● *Treponema pallidum* haemagglutination (TPHA) test.
● *Treponema pallidum* particle agglutination (TPPA) test.
● Treponemal enzyme immunoassay (EIA).

Treatment
● Procaine penicillin G, doxycycline, erythromycin, azithromycin.
● N.B. If the patient has neurosyphilis then give them prophylactic prednisolone to avoid the Jarisch–Herxheimer reaction. This reaction may occur after antibacterial treatment, which causes the death of the spirochaete and subsequent endotoxin release. Endotoxins cause the Jarisch–Herxheimer reaction.

MAP 7.5 **Sexually Transmitted Infections (STIs)**

Complications
- Gumma formation.
- Meningitis.
- Stroke.
- Heart valve damage.

CHLAMYDIA TRACHOMATIS
What is *Chlamydia trachomatis*?
This is an Gram-negative bacterium that causes chlamydia.

Investigations
- Chlamydia cell culture.
- Nucleic acid amplification test (NAAT).
- Direct fluorescent antibody test (DFA).

Treatment
- Azithromycin (single dose) or doxycycline (for 7 days).

Complications
- Pelvic inflammatory disease.
- Urethritis.
- Infertility.
- Postpartum endometritis.

Remember 3Hs
- **Hepatitis** see page 46.
- **Herpes** see page 110.
- **HIV** see page 112.

NEISSERIA GONORRHOEAE
What is *Neisseria gonorrhoeae*?
This is a Gram-negative diplococcus that causes gonorrhoea.
It is sometimes asymptomatic or presents with discharge.

Investigations
- NAAT.
- Cultured on chocolate agar.

Treatment
- Azithromycin (single dose) and ceftriaxone (single dose).

Complications
- Pelvic inflammatory disease.
- Infertility.
- Dissemination of bacteria.

Map 7.5 Sexually Transmitted Infections (STIs)

Infectious Disease

Map 7.6 Bacterial Infections

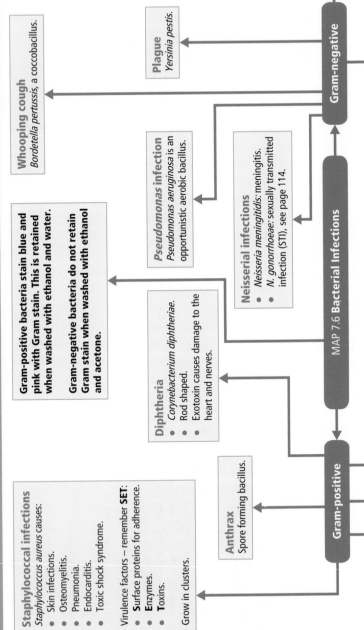

Staphylococcal infections
Staphylococcus aureus causes:
- Skin infections.
- Osteomyelitis.
- Pneumonia.
- Endocarditis.
- Toxic shock syndrome.

Virulence factors – remember **SET**:
- **S**urface proteins for adherence.
- **E**nzymes.
- **T**oxins.

Grow in clusters.

Anthrax
Spore forming bacillus.

Diphtheria
- *Corynebacterium diphtheriae*.
- Rod shaped.
- Exotoxin causes damage to the heart and nerves.

Gram-positive bacteria stain blue and pink when washed with Gram stain. This is retained when washed with ethanol and water.

Gram-negative bacteria do not retain Gram stain when washed with ethanol and acetone.

Pseudomonas infection
Pseudomonas aeruginosa is an opportunistic aerobic bacillus.

Neisserial infections
- *Neisseria meningitidis*: meningitis.
- *N. gonorrhoeae*: sexually transmitted infection (STI), see page 114.

Whooping cough
Bordetella pertussis, a coccobacillus.

Plague
Yersinia pestis.

Gram-negative

MAP 7.6 **Bacterial Infections**

Gram-positive

Granuloma inguinale
- *Klebsiella granulomatis.*
- An encapsulated coccobacillus.
- Causes ulcerative genital infection.

Chancroid
- *Haemophilus ducreyi.*
- Causes ulcerative genital infection.

Nocardia
- *Nocardia asteroides.*
- Aerobic.
- Grows in branched chains.
- Causes opportunistic respiratory infections with central nervous system involvement.

Listeriosis
- *Listeria monocytogenes.*
- Facultative intracellular bacillus.
- Causes meningitis in the elderly and immunosuppressed.

Streptococcal infections
- Facultative or obligate anaerobes.
- *Streptococcus pneumoniae:* acquired pneumonia, see page 20 and meningitis.
- Enterococci: urinary tract infection and endocarditis.

Virulence factors:
- Capsules, which resist phagocytosis.
- M protein, which inhibits the alternative pathway of the complement system.
- Pneumolysin, which destroys the membranes of host cells.

Grow in pairs or chains.

Map 7.6 Bacterial Infections

Map 7.7 Viral Infections

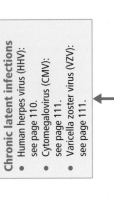

MAP 7.7 Viral Infections

Chronic latent infections
- Human herpes virus (HHV): see page 110.
- Cytomegalovirus (CMV): see page 111.
- Varicella zoster virus (VZV): see page 111.

TRANSIENT INFECTIONS

Rhinovirus
- Enterovirus.
- Causes the common cold.

Influenza
- RNA virus.
- Causes the flu.
- Classified into 3 types: A, B and C.

Polio virus
- Unencapsulated RNA enterovirus.

Measles
- RNA paramyxovirus.
- Host cells develop T cell-mediated immunity to control this viral infection.
- Rash is caused by hypersensitivity to the viral antigens within the skin.

Mumps
- Paramyxovirus.
- Causes inflammation of the parotid glands.
- Sometimes travels to central nervous system (CNS), pancreas and testes.

West Nile virus
- Arthropod virus of the flavivirus group.
- Invades the CNS causing meningitis and encephalitis.
- Seen in the elderly and immunosuppressed.

TRANSFORMING INFECTIONS

Human immunodeficiency virus (HIV)
See page 112.

Human papillomavirus (HPV)
This is associated with cervical cancer (this is because the HPV E6 and HPV E7 gene products dysregulate the cell cycle).

Epstein–Barr virus (EBV)
- Causes infectious mononucleosis.
- Usually self-limiting.
- Presents with fever and sore throat.
- Associated with Burkitt's lymphoma (8;14 translocation of *c-myc* oncogene), see page 102.

Chronic productive infections
- Hepatitis virus, see page 46.

Map 7.7 Viral Infections

Map 7.8 Vaccines

DNA vaccines

- Potentially in the future.
- Usually a harmless virus which has a gene for a protective antigen spliced into it.
- This protective antigen is generated within the vaccine recipient and elicits an immune response.

Advantages:

- Plasmids are easily manufactured and do not replicate.
- DNA is stable and sequencing may be changed.
- Temperature extremes are resisted; therefore, it is easily transported and stored.
- Cheap.

Disadvantages:

- Plasmids could integrate into the host genome.
- Immunological tolerance.

Subunit

- E.g. hepatitis B, tetanus, diphtheria.
- This is a vaccine containing purified components of the virus.
- Example components include the surface antigen.

MAP 7.8 **Vaccines**

Inactivated

- E.g. polio (Salk), rabies, hepatitis A, influenza.
- Preparations of the wild type virus.
- The virus is nonpathogenic because of chemical treatment (e.g. with formalin).
- This chemical treatment cross-links viral proteins.

Advantages:
- Sufficient humoral immunity if boosters given.
- Good for immunosuppressed patients.
- No mutations of virus.
- Good for those living in tropical areas.

Disadvantages:
- Some do not increase immunity.
- Boosters are required.
- Expensive.
- Potential failure of viral inactivation process.
- Little local immunity.

Attenuated

- E.g. polio (Sabin), mumps, measles, rubella (MMR), varicella, rotavirus, yellow fever.
- Live virus particles grow in the vaccine recipient.
- However, these particles do not cause disease because the virus has been mutated to a form that is nonpathogenic, e.g. the virus tropism has been altered.

Advantages:
- Activates all phases of the immune system.
- It stimulates antibodies against multiple epitopes.
- Provides cheap and fast immunity.
- It has the potential to eliminate the wild type virus from the community.
- Easily transported.

Disadvantages:
- If the mutation fails then the virus will revert to its virulent form.
- Potential spread of the mutated viral form.
- Do NOT give to immunocompromised patients.
- Not good for those living in tropical areas.

Chapter Eight The Immune System

The Immune System

Map 8.1 Cells of the Immune System

Dendritic cells
- Antigen presenting cells.
- In skin they are referred to as Langerhans cells.

Myeloid progenitor cells

Mast cells
- Involved in allergic reactions.
- Degranulate producing histamine, heparin and chemotactic factors (for eosinophils).

Leucocytes

MAP 8.1 **Cells of the Immune System**

Lymphocytes

T lymphocytes
- Arise from bone marrow but mature in thymus.
- Different types:
  - Cytotoxic CD8+ cells.
  - Helper CD4+ cells.
  - Suppressor cells.

B lymphocytes
- Part of the humoral immune system.
- Arise from bone marrow and mature there.

Plasma cells

- B cells differentiate into plasma cells when they come across an antigen.
- Plasma cells produce specific antibodies.

Myeloblasts

Granulocytes

Basophils
- Allergic reactions.
- Bilobate nucleus.

Eosinophils
- Bilobate nucleus.
- In allergic reactions and parasite infections.

Neutrophils
- Acute inflammatory response.
- Multilobed nucleus.

Monocytes
- Kidney shaped nucleus.
- Differentiate into macrophages.

Macrophages
- Phagocytic.
- Scavenger cells: they scavenge and destroy.
- γ-interferon activates macrophages.

Map 8.1 Cells of the Immune System

The Immune System

The Immune System

Map 8.2 Antibodies

MAP 8.2 **Antibodies**

IgA
- Dimer (when secreted).
- Prevents bacteria and viruses from attaching to and colonising mucosal surfaces.
- Found in colostrum, breast milk, saliva, mucosal surfaces and tears.

IgD
- Monomer.
- Activates basophils.
- Activates mast cells.

IgM
- Pentamer (when secreted).
- Fixes complement.
- Involved in primary immune response.

IgG
- Monomer.
- Only immunoglobulin to cross the placenta.
- Involved in secondary immune response.
- Largest concentration of immunoglobulin in the blood.
- Fixes complement system.

IgE
- Monomer.
- Binds to allergens and causes mast cells to degranulate. This results in histamine release.
- Binds to basophils, also causing histamine release.
- Activates eosinophils.
- IgE plays a role in protection against parasitic worm infection.

MAP 8.3 **The Complement System**

Part of the innate immune system

Consists of 3 pathways
Remember **CAL**:
- **C**lassical complement pathway.
- **A**lternative complement pathway.
- **L**ectin complement pathway.

Functions
Remember **COCA**:
- **C**hemotaxis.
- **O**psonisation.
- **C**ell lysis.
- **A**ntigen bearing agents are clumped together.

The Immune System

Map 8.4 Activation of the Complement System

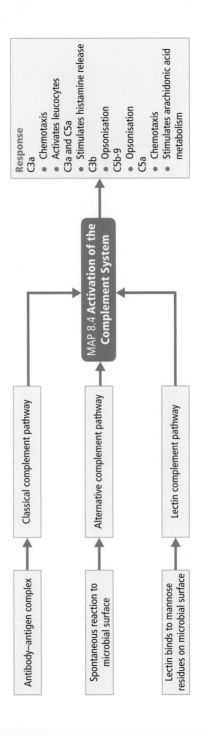

Response

C3a
- Chemotaxis
- Activates leucocytes

C3a and C5a
- Stimulates histamine release

C3b
- Opsonisation

C5b-9
- Opsonisation

C5a
- Chemotaxis
- Stimulates arachidonic acid metabolism

MAP 8.4 **Activation of the Complement System**

Classical complement pathway

Alternative complement pathway

Lectin complement pathway

Antibody–antigen complex

Spontaneous reaction to microbial surface

Lectin binds to mannose residues on microbial surface

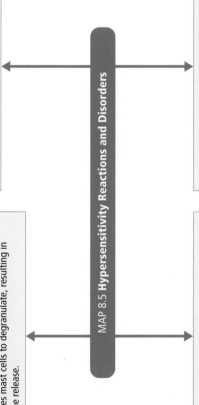

Type I (immediate hypersensitivity)
- E.g. Hay fever, allergic reaction to a wasp sting.
- Anaphylactic reaction.
- IgE involvement.
- Antigen presents to CD4+ cells, which stimulates IgE production.
- IgE causes mast cells to degranulate, resulting in histamine release.

Type II (cytotoxic hypersensitivity)
- E.g. Graves' disease, see page 72, myasthenia gravis, rheumatic fever.
- Antibody-mediated reaction.
- IgM, IgG and complement (classical pathway) involvement.

MAP 8.5 Hypersensitivity Reactions and Disorders

Type III (immune-complex reactions)
- E.g. Systemic lupus erythematosus, see page 130, rheumatoid arthritis, see page 157.
- Immune complex reaction.
- IgG and complement involvement.

Type IV (delayed hypersensitivity)
- E.g. Hashimoto's thyroiditis, see page 74, multiple sclerosis, see page 153.
- Cell-mediated reaction.
- T cell involvement.

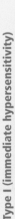

Map 8.6 Systemic Lupus Erythematosus (SLE)

Investigations

- Antinuclear antibody (ANA).
- Anti-Smith antibodies and antidouble-stranded DNA.
- Bloods: FBC, U&Es, LFTs, TFTs, glucose.
- GFR: assessment of renal function.
- Pulmonary function tests.

What is SLE?

SLE is a multisystemic autoimmune disease that usually affects females of childbearing age.

Causes

The exact cause of SLE is unknown. It is thought to be an autoimmune reaction in genetically susceptible individuals.

Signs and symptoms

- Fatigue.
- Myalgia.
- Rashes: malar (butterfly) rash, discoid rash.
- Raynaud's phenomenon.
- Arthritis.
- Central nervous system disorders: epilepsy, headache.
- Haematological disorders: haemolytic anaemia.
- Immunological disorders.
- Nephritis.
- Oral ulcers.
- Photosensitivity.
- Pericarditis.
- Pleuritis.

MAP 8.6 **Systemic Lupus Erythematosus (SLE)**

Complications

- Increased risk of atherosclerosis.
- Increased risk of stroke.
- Increased risk of myocardial infarction.
- Risk of lupus nephritis.
- Increased risk of other autoimmune conditions.
- Depression.

Revised criteria for diagnosing SLE

≥4/11 is diagnostic. Remember this as
I AM PORN HSD:

- **I**mmunological disorder.

- **A**NA positive.
- **M**alar rash.

- **P**hotosensitivity.
- **O**ral ulcers.
- **R**enal disorder.
- **N**onerosive arthritis, **N**eurological disorder.

- **H**aematological disorder.
- **S**erositis.
- **D**iscoid rash.

Treatment

- Conservative: patient education. Advise patient about sun protection and encourage smoking cessation. Assess psychological impact of disease.
- Medical:
  - Analgesia (nonsteroidal anti-inflammatory drugs).
  - Steroid therapy.
  - Immunosuppressive therapy, e.g. azathioprine, cyclophosphamide.
  - Monoclonal antibodies, e.g. rituximab.

Map 8.6 Systemic Lupus Erythematosus (SLE)

Map 9.1 Regions of the Brain

Frontal lobe
- Is responsible for motor control of the opposite side of the body, e.g. the left frontal lobe has motor control of the right side of the body.
- Controls emotion and insight.
- The dominant hemisphere is responsible for speech output (Broca's area).
- Primary motor cortex: located in the posterior portion of the frontal lobe. This area plans and executes movement.
- Broca's area: located in the frontal lobe, just superior to the lateral fissure. It is responsible for the formation of speech.

Basal ganglia
- Is an interconnection of deep nuclei:
  o Putamen and globus pallidus: together they form the lentiform nucleus.
  o Caudate nucleus.
  o Substantia nigra.
  o Subthalamic nucleus.
- Integrates motor and sensory inputs.

Parietal lobe
- Is responsible for sensation of the opposite side of the body.
- It is also responsible for spatial awareness.
- Somatosensory cortex: located in the anterior cortex of the parietal lobe. It processes pain, pressure and touch.

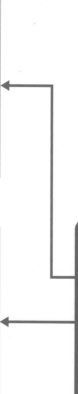

MAP 9.1 **Regions of the Brain**

Occipital lobe
- Is responsible for vision.
- Primary visual cortex is located within this lobe.

Temporal lobe
- Is responsible for memory and emotion.
- In the dominant hemisphere it is responsible for the comprehension of speech (Wernicke's area).
- Wernicke's area: allows spoken and written language to be comprehended. It is located just posterior to the superior temporal gyrus.
- Primary auditory complex: responsible for hearing. It is located within the temporal lobe bilaterally.

Cerebellum
This is split into 3 lobes:
1 The paleocerebellum: maintains gait.
2 The neocerebellum: maintains postural tone and is responsible for the co-ordination of fine motor skills.
3 The archicerebellum: maintains balance.

FIGURE 9.1 **The Blood Supply of the Brain**

Circle of Willis

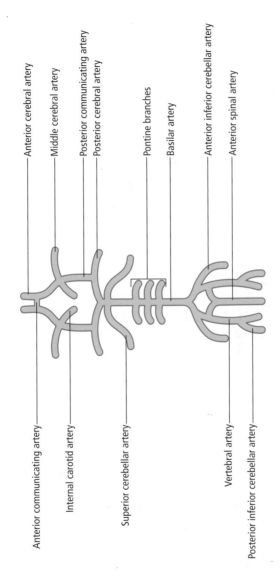

Anterior cerebral artery

Middle cerebral artery

Posterior communicating artery

Posterior cerebral artery

Pontine branches

Basilar artery

Anterior inferior cerebellar artery

Anterior spinal artery

Anterior communicating artery

Internal carotid artery

Superior cerebellar artery

Vertebral artery

Posterior inferior cerebellar artery

Figure 9.1 The Blood Supply of the Brain

Table 9.1 The Cranial Nerves and their Lesions

TABLE 9.1 The Cranial Nerves and their Lesions

Nerve	Sensory or motor	Location	Function	Lesion
I: Olfactory	Sensory	Cribriform plate of the ethmoid bone	Sense of smell	Loss of smell (anosmia)
II: Optic	Sensory	Optic canal	Sight	Different visual field losses depending on the location of the lesion
III: Oculomotor	Motor	Superior orbital fissure	Innervates the superior, medial and inferior rectus muscles as well as the levator palpebrae superioris, inferior oblique and sphincter pupillae	Eye moves down and out due to unopposed action of the superior oblique and lateral rectus muscles; ptosis (drooping eyelid) and mydriasis (dilated pupil) are observed
IV: Trochlear	Motor	Superior orbital fissure	Innervates the superior oblique muscle	Diplopia and eye moves down and in
V: Trigeminal	Motor and sensory	V1: ophthalmic nerve: superior orbital fissure V2: maxillary nerve: foramen rotundum V3: mandibular nerve: foramen ovale	Sensation of the face and innervates the muscles of mastication; test corneal reflex	Decreased facial sensation and jaw weakness
VI: Abducens	Motor	Superior orbital fissure	Innervates the lateral rectus muscle	Eye deviates medially

VII: Facial	Motor and sensory	Internal acoustic canal and exits through the stylomastoid foramen	Innervates the muscles of facial expression, stapedius, posterior belly of the digastric muscle, stylohyoid, taste anterior 2/3 tongue, the lacrimal gland and the salivary glands (not parotids)	Upper motor neuron (UMN): asymmetry of lower face with forehead sparing Lower motor neuron (LMN): asymmetry of upper and lower face; loss of taste, hyperacusis and eye irritation due to ↓ lacrimation
VIII: Vestibulocochlear	Sensory	Internal acoustic canal	Sense of sound and balance	Deafness and vertigo
IX: Glossopharyngeal	Motor and sensory	Jugular foramen	Supplies taste to posterior 1/3 tongue and innervates the parotids as well as the stylopharyngeus	Decreased gag reflex, uvular deviation away from lesion
X: Vagus	Motor and sensory	Jugular foramen	Innervates laryngeal and pharyngeal muscles (not stylopharyngeus) and parasympathetic supply to thoracic and abdominal viscera	Dysphagia, recurrent laryngeal nerve palsies and pseudobulbar palsies
XI: spinal Accessory	Motor	Jugular foramen	Innervates trapezius and sternocleidomastoid muscles	Patient cannot shrug and displays weak head movement
XII: Hypoglossal	Motor	Hypoglossal canal	Innervates the muscles of the tongue (except for the palatoglossal, which is supplied by the vagus nerve)	Tongue deviates towards the side of weakness during protrusion

Table 9.1 The Cranial Nerves and their Lesions

Figure 9.2 Ascending and Descending Spinal Pathways

FIGURE 9.2 **Ascending and Descending Spinal Pathways**

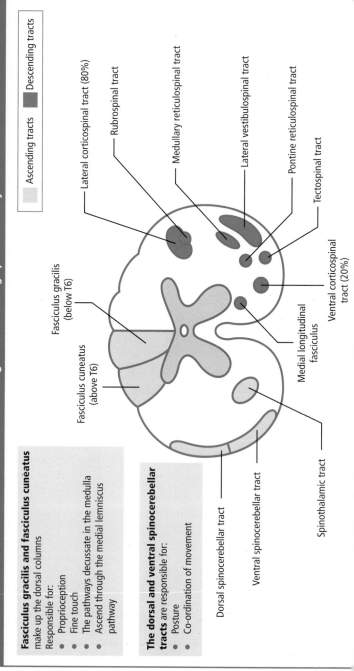

Ascending tracts — Descending tracts

Lateral corticospinal tract (80%)

Rubrospinal tract

Medullary reticulospinal tract

Lateral vestibulospinal tract

Pontine reticulospinal tract

Tectospinal tract

Ventral corticospinal tract (20%)

Medial longitudinal fasciculus

Spinothalamic tract

Ventral spinocerebellar tract

Dorsal spinocerebellar tract

Fasciculus cuneatus (above T6)

Fasciculus gracilis (below T6)

Fasciculus gracilis and fasciculus cuneatus
make up the dorsal columns
Responsible for:
- Proprioception
- Fine touch
- The pathways decussate in the medulla
- Ascend through the medial lemniscus pathway

The dorsal and ventral spinocerebellar tracts are responsible for:
- Posture
- Co-ordination of movement

Dorsal spinocerebellar tract
- Originates from Clarke's column
- Location: inferior cerebellar peduncle
- Ipsilateral

Ventral spinocerebellar tract
- Location: superior cerebellar peduncle
- Contralateral

Spinothalamic tract
- Decussate at level of entry
- Anterior: crude touch
- Posterior: pain and temperature
Responsible for:
- Pain
- Pressure
- Nondiscriminative touch

Lateral corticospinal tract (80%)
- Voluntary skilled movements at the DISTAL parts of limbs

Tectospinal tract
- Originates in the superior colliculus
Responsible for:
- Reflective movements of the head in response to visual/auditory stimuli

Rubrospinal tract
- Location: red nucleus of the midbrain
- Afferent fibres are received from the cerebellum and motor cortex
Responsible for:
- Control of limb flexor muscles

Medullary reticulospinal tract
- Bilateral
Responsible for:
- Reflex activity
- Control of breathing
- Control of alpha and gamma neurons

Lateral vestibulospinal tract
- From vestibular nucleus in pons and medulla
Responsible for:
- EXTENSOR muscle tone
- Posture

Pontine reticulospinal tract
- Ipsilateral

Figure 9.2 Ascending and Descending Spinal Pathways

Map 9.2 Stroke

Investigations

- Bloods: FBC, U&Es, LFTs, PTT, glucose, cholesterol levels.
- Other: ECG for AF and ECHO for structural abnormalities. Glascow Coma Scale to assess level of consciousness.
- Radiology: CT head and diffusion-weighted MRI (DWI) immediately if any indication of stroke. It is important to distinguish between haemorrhagic and ischaemic stroke since treatment options differ.

Risk factors

- ↑ Blood pressure.
- Atrial fibrillation (AF).
- Diabetes mellitus.
- Smoking.
- Alcohol.
- Previous stroke.
- The oral contraceptive pill.
- Disorder that increases clotting.
- Cocaine use.
- ↑ Cholesterol.

Complications

- Hydrocephalus.
- Increased risk of deep vein thrombosis (DVT).
- Aphasia.
- Dysphagia.
- Decreased muscle movement.
- Amnesia.
- Depression.

MAP 9.2 **Stroke**

What is a stroke?

A stroke is a vascular insult to the brain causing a focal neurological deficit. This occurs due to ischaemic infarct or haemorrhage, which disrupts the blood supply to the brain.

Signs and symptoms

These vary depending on the circulation affected by the infarct or haemorrhage.

Acute signs and symptoms may be remembered as **FAST**:

- **Face:** unilateral drooping.
- **Arms:** these may feel weak and numb. Patient may not be able to lift them.
- **Speech:** slurring of speech.
- **Time:** time for emergency medical attention, call 999 (UK) immediately.

Stroke may also be associated with transient ischaemic attack (TIA). This is a focal neurological deficit where symptoms last <24 h due to temporary occlusion of the cerebral circulation. Patients may describe amaurosis fugax – loss of sight described as 'curtains descending'. The phenomenon lasts <24 h and is usually followed by stroke within 90 days.

Causes

- Haemorrhagic causes:
  - Central nervous system bleeds from trauma.
  - Ruptured aneurysm.
- Ishcaemic causes:
  - Small vessel occlusion.
  - Atherothromboembolism.
  - Cardiac emboli.
  - Emboli secondary to AF.

Treatment

- Conservative: patient and family education, initiate early mobilisation, commence stroke rehabilitation, assess speech and swallowing. Assess impact of activities of daily living (ADLs) using Barthel index.
- Medical:
  - TIA patients:
    - Assess risk of subsequent stroke using ABCD2 (high risk is a score >6, low risk is a score <4). ABCD2: **A**ge >60 years (1 point); **B**lood pressure >140/90 mmHg (1 point); **C**linical features: unilateral weakness (2 points), isolated speech disturbance (1 point); **D**uration of symptoms: >60 min (2 points), 10–59 min (1 point); **D**iabetes (1 point).
    - Start aspirin 300 mg.
  - Ischaemic stroke patients without haemorrhage:
    - Thrombolysis with alteplase within 3 h (patients >80 years) and within 4.5 h (patients <80 years).
    - Start aspirin 300 mg (unless contraindications).
  - Haemorrhagic stroke patients:
    - Prothrombin complex concentrate.
    - Intravenous vitamin K.
- Surgical:
  - Referral for acute intracerebral haemorrhage.
  - Referral for decompressive hemicraniectomy.

Map 9.2 Stroke

TABLE 9.2 Dementia

This is a syndrome of a progressive global decline in cognitive function

Type of dementia	Causes	Signs and symptoms	Investigations	Treatment	Complications
Alzheimer's disease	Exact cause unknown Risk factors include: • ↑ *APP* gene load • Down's syndrome due to • Familial gene associations: ○ Amyloid precursor protein (APP): chromosome 21 ○ Presenilin-1: chromosome 14 ○ Presenilin-2: chromosome 1 ○ Apolipoprotein E4 (ApoE4) alleles: chromosome 19 • Hypothyroidism • Previous head trauma • Family history of Alzheimer's disease	Amnesia Disorientation Changes in personality Decreasing self care Apraxia Agnosia Aphasia Lexical anomia Paranoid delusions Depression Wandering Aggression Sexual disinhibition	Mental state examination Addenbrooke's Cognitive Examination (ACE-III) Bloods: FBC, U&Es, LFTs, TFTs, CRP, ESR, glucose, calcium, magnesium, phosphate, VDRL, HIV serology, vitamin B_{12} and folate levels, blood culture, ECG, lumbar puncture, CXR, CT scan, MRI scan, SPECT 3 main findings on histology – **BAT:** • **B**eta amyloid plaques • ↓ **A**cetylcholine • neurofibrillary **T**angles	Memantine: inhibits glutamate by blocking N-methyl-D-aspartate (NMDA) receptors Donepezil: acetylcholinesterase inhibitor Rivastigmine: acetylcholinesterase inhibitor	Amnesia Increased risk of infection Dysphagia Urinary incontinence Increased risk of falls
Vascular dementia	Is the second most common cause of dementia It is caused by infarcts of small and medium sized vessels in the brain Genetic association with	It follows a deteriorating stepwise progression. There are 3 types: 1 Vascular dementia following stroke 2 Multi-infarct dementia	Mental state examination ACE-III Bloods: FBC, U&Es, LFTs, TFTs, CRP, ESR, glucose, calcium, magnesium, phosphate,	Dietary advice Smoking cessation Treat diabetes mellitus and hypertension Aspirin	Significant co-morbidity, e.g. cardiovascular disease and renal disease

Table 9.2 Dementia

	cerebral autosomal dominant arteriopathy with subcortical infarcts and leucoencephalopathy (CADASIL) on chromosome 19	following multiple strokes 3 Binswanger disease following microvascular infarcts Amnesia Disorientation Changes in personality Decreasing self care Depression Signs of upper motor neuron (UMN) lesions, e.g. brisk reflexes Seizures	VDRL, HIV serology, vitamin B_{12} and folate levels, cholesterol levels, vasculitis screen, syphilis serology ECG, lumbar puncture, CXR, CT scan, MRI scan, SPECT		
Dementia with Lewy bodies	Associated with Parkinson's disease Avoid antipsychotic drugs in these patients	Is a triad of: 1 Parkinsonism: bradykinesia, gait disorder 2 Hallucinations: predominantly visual hallucinations, usually of animals and people 3 Disease process follows a fluctuating course	Mental state examination ACE-III CT scan, MRI scan, SPECT scan ApoE genotype Lewy bodies, ubiquitin proteins and alpha-synuclein found on histology	AVOID ANTIPSYCHOTICS: causes hypersensitivity to neuroleptics Levodopa may be used to treat Parkinson's symptoms but these may worsen psychotic symptoms	Neuroleptic hypersensitivity Autonomic dysfunction Fluctuating blood pressure Arrhythmias Urinary incontinence Dysphagia Increased risk of falls

Continued overleaf

Table 9.2 Dementia

TABLE 9.2 **Dementia** (*Continued*)

This is a syndrome of a progressive global decline in cognitive function

Type of dementia	Causes	Signs and symptoms	Investigations	Treatment	Complications
Frontotemporal dementia (Pick's disease)	Genetic association with chromosome 17q21 – 22 and tau 3 gene mutations	Amnesia Disorientation Changes in personality Decreasing self care Mutism Echolalia Overeating Parkinsonism Disinhibition	Mental state examination ACE-III CT scan, MRI scan, SPECT scan Histology – depends on subtype: • Microvacuolar type: microvacuolation • Pick type: widespread gliosis, no microvacuolation • Motor neuron disease (MND) type: histological changes like MND	Currently none. Only supportive treatment available	Increased risk of falls Increased risk of infection
Huntington's dementia	A complication of Huntington's disease (see page 204), which is an autosomal dominant disorder where there is a defective gene on chromosome 4 Causes uncontrollable choreiform movements and dementia	Uncontrollable choreiform movements Depression Irritability Anxiety Psychosis Obsessive compulsive behaviour	Diagnostic genetic testing	No cure. Treat symptoms: • Chorea: an atypical antipsychotic agent • Obsessive compulsive thoughts and irritability: selective serotonin reuptake inhibitors (SSRIs)	Dysphagia Increased risk of falls Increased risk of infection

Table 9.2 Dementia

Creutzfeldt–Jakob disease (CJD)	Caused by prions Progressive and without cure There is also variant CJD (vCJD), which has an earlier onset of death	Rapidly progressive dementia (4–5 months) Amnesia Disorientation Changes in personality Depression Psychosis Ataxia Seizures	EEG: triphasic spikes seen Lumbar puncture (LP): for 14-3-3 protein CT scan MRI scan	No cure	Increased risk of infection Coma Heart failure Respiratory failure
Other causes	HIV Vitamin B_{12} deficiency Syphilis Wilson's disease: autosomal recessive condition where copper accumulates within the tissues Dementia pugilistica: seen in boxers and patients who suffer multiple concussions; also known as 'punch drunk' syndrome				

Table 9.2 Dementia

Map 9.3 Epilepsy

What is epilepsy?

This is a condition in which the brain is affected by recurrent seizures. These seizures may be defined in many different ways:

- Partial seizures: this is a seizure that occurs in one discrete part of the brain. These seizures may be simple (without alteration in consciousness) or complex (with alteration in consciousness).
- Generalised seizures: these seizures affect the brain globally. Consciousness is always altered. Examples include:
  o Absence seizures: often picked up in children who 'stare into space'. The seizure usually only lasts seconds.
  o Tonic–clonic seizures: involves convulsions and muscle rigidity. Usually last minutes.
  o Atonic seizures: involves a loss of muscle tone.
  o Myotonic: involves jerky muscle movements.
  o Secondary generalised: this is a generalised seizure that originates from a partial seizure.

Investigations

- Bloods: FBC, U&Es, LFTs, CRP, ESR, glucose, calcium levels.
- Radiology: CT scan, MRI scan.
- Other: ECG, LP, EEG.

Signs and symptoms

These depend on the region of the brain affected.

- Frontal lobe, remember **JAM:**
  o **J**acksonian march.
  o **pA**lsy (postictal Todd's palsy).
  o **M**otor features.
- Temporal lobe, remember **ADD FAT:**
  o **A**ura that the epileptic attack will occur.
  o **D**éjà vu.
  o **D**elusional behaviour.
  o **F**ear/panic: hippocampal involvement.
  o **A**utomatisms.
  o **T**aste/smell: uncal involvement.
- Parietal and occipital lobe: visual and sensory disturbances.
- Others include: partial or generalised seizure with or without convulsions, tongue biting, migraines and depression.

MAP 9.3 **Epilepsy**

Causes

Seizures are caused by abnormal paroxysmal neuronal discharges in the brain, which are usually a result of some form of traumatic brain injury. These discharges display hypersynchronisation. The causes of epilepsy may be broadly classified into 3 types:

1 Idiopathic: cause for epilepsy is unknown.
2 Cryptogenic: cause for epilepsy is unknown, but there are signs suggesting it may be linked to brain injury, e.g. patient has autism or learning difficulties.
3 Symptomatic: cause known. Some causes of symptomatic epilepsy include:

VINDICATE:

○ **V**ascular: history of stroke.
○ **I**nfection: history of meningitis or malaria.
○ **N**eoplasms: brain tumour.
○ **D**rugs: alcohol and illicit drug use.
○ **I**atrogenic: drug withdrawal.
○ **C**ongenital: family history of epilepsy.
○ **A**utoimmune: vasculitis.
○ **T**rauma: history of brain injury.
○ **E**ndocrine: ↓ Na$^+$, ↓ Ca^{2+}, ↓ or ↑ glucose.

Complications

- Injuries whilst having seizure.
- Depression.
- Anxiety.
- Brain damage.
- Sudden unexplained death in epilepsy (SUDEP).

Treatment

- Conservative: patient and family education. Inform DVLA (UK).
- Medical: anticonvulsant therapy, see Table 9.3.
- Surgical: anterior temporal lobe resection, corpus callosotomy, tumour removal.

Map 9.3   Epilepsy

TABLE 9.3 Anticonvulsant Drugs

N.B. for a full description of epilepsy management and which drugs to use as first line, please follow the website link provided for NICE guidelines (Appendix 2)

Anticonvulsant agent	Mechanism of action	Uses	Side-effects	Contraindications	Drug interactions
Carbamazepine	Blocks voltage dependent Na+ channels	All seizures except absence seizures Neuropathic pain, e.g. trigeminal neuralgia Manic–depressive illness	Rash Sedation Drowsiness Hyponatraemia Dry mouth Blurring of vision Neutropenia Hallucinations	Pregnancy (it is teratogenic) Past history of bone marrow depression Acute porphyria	Alters metabolism of oral contraceptive pill Alters metabolism of warfarin Alters metabolism of corticosteroids
Phenytoin	Blocks voltage dependent Na+ channels	All seizures except pure absence seizures Seizure prevention post neurosurgery Trigeminal neuralgia Arrhythmia Digoxin toxicity	Rash Hypersensitivity reactions Ataxia Megaloblastic anaemia Hirsutism Gum hypertrophy Purple glove syndrome	Pregnancy (it is teratogenic) Sinus bradycardia Stokes–Adams syndrome Sinoatrial block Second degree heart block Third degree heart block	Sodium valproate alters (increases or decreases) phenytoin concentration Phenytoin increases metabolism of drugs like anticoagulants by enzyme induction Phenytoin reduces concentration of mirtazapine N.B. This drug has a narrow therapeutic index

Table 9.3 Anticonvulsant Drugs

	Mechanism	Indications	Side effects	Contraindications	Interactions
Sodium valproate	Blocks voltage dependent Na$^+$ channels Weakly inhibits gamma-amino butyric acid (GABA) transaminase	All seizures Anxiety disorders Anorexia nervosa Manic–depressive illness	Nausea Vomiting Weight gain Hair loss Thinning of hair Curling of hair Hepatotoxicity Tremor Parkinsonism Thrombocytopenia Encephalopathy	Pregnancy (it is teratogenic) Hepatic failure History of mitochondrial disease	Aspirin increases levels of sodium valproate Sodium valproate may enhance effects of anticoagulant coumarins Carbamazepine decreases levels of sodium valproate
Ethosuximide	Inhibits T-type Ca^{2+} channels	Absence seizures (used more frequently in children)	Nausea Vomiting Anorexia Hypersensitivity reactions Blood dyscrasias Ataxia	Pregnancy (it is teratogenic) Hepatic failure Affective disorders Systemic lupus erythematosus	Metabolism is inhibited by isoniazid Sodium valproate increases the level of ethosuximide Phenytoin and carbamazepine decrease the level of ethosuximide
Phenobarbital	Acts on GABA$_A$ receptors, enhancing synaptic inhibition	All seizures except absence seizures Status epilepticus (third line) Anaesthesia Neonatal seizures Cyclical vomiting syndrome Crigler–Najjar syndrome Gilbert syndrome	Rash Sedation Depression Ataxia Amelogenesis imperfecta	Pregnancy (it is teratogenic) History of porphyria	Phenobarbital increases metabolism of coumarins Carbamazepine increases concentration of phenobarbital Phenobarbital decreases levels of itraconazole

Continued overleaf

Table 9.3 Anticonvulsant Drugs

TABLE 9.3 **Anticonvulsant Drugs** (*Continued*)

N.B. for a full description of epilepsy management and which drugs to use as first line, please follow the website link provided for NICE guidelines (Appendix 2)

Anticonvulsant agent	Mechanism of action	Uses	Side-effects	Contraindications	Drug interactions
Benzodiazepines	Allosterically modifies GABA$_A$ receptor, thereby increasing Cl$^-$ conductance	Lorazepam used to treat status epilepticus (first line) Anxiety disorders Insomnia Seizures Alcohol withdrawal	Sedation Withdrawal syndrome Respiratory depression	Chronic obstructive pulmonary disease Sleep apnoea Myasthenia gravis Severe depression (increased suicidal tendencies)	Use cautiously with other central nervous system depressants, e.g. opioids and barbiturates Increasing sedative effect when used with antihistamines Increasing sedative effect when used with antipsychotics
Vigabatrin	Inhibits GABA transaminase	All seizures Seizures in patients who are resistant to other anticonvulsant medication	Sedation Headache Peripheral visual field defect Depression Psychosis Hallucinations	Hypersensitivity	Vigabatrin increases clearance of carbamazepine Vigabatrin decreases levels of phenytoin

Table 9.3 Anticonvulsant Drugs

Lamotrigine	Blocks voltage dependent Na$^+$ channels Inhibits L-, N- and P-type Ca^{2+} channels	All seizures Manic–depressive illness Severedepression Neuropathic pain, e.g. trigeminal neuralgia	Stevens–Johnson syndrome Toxic epidermal necrolysis (Lyell's syndrome) Rashes Nausea Ataxia	Hypersensitivity Hepatic failure	The oral contraceptive pill decreases levels of lamotrigine Carbemazepine decreases lamotrigine levels Rifampicin decreases levels of lamotrigine Valproate increases levels of lamotrigine
Gabapentin and pregabalin	Gapapentin is a GABA analogue Pregabalin is an analogue of gabapentin	All seizures Neuropathic pain Manic–depressive illness	Sedation Ataxia	Hypersensitivity	When used with propoxyphene patients are more at risk of side-effects such as dizziness and confusion Bioavailability of gabapentin increased by morphine

Table 9.3 Anticonvulsant Drugs

Map 9.4 Parkinson's Disease

What is Parkinson's disease?

This is a progressive disorder of the central nervous system, which is due to dopamine depletion.

Causes

The exact cause of this degenerative disease is unknown but some postulated risk factors include:

- Male gender.
- Genetic component.
- Environmental exposure to insecticides, pesticides and herbicides.

Pathophysiology

- ↓ Dopamine producing cells in the pars compacta region of the substantia nigra, located in the midbrain.
- Dopamine produced is secreted to the putamen and caudate nucleus.
- ↑ Lewy bodies in the substantia nigra.

Signs and symptoms

Remember **Facial TRAPS**:

- **Facial:** expressionless face.
- **Tremor** (pill rolling tremor).
- **Rigidity** (cog wheel rigidity).
- **Akinesia.**
- **Posture** (stooped).
- **Shuffling gait.**

Investigations

There is no specific test for Parkinson's disease. It is a clinical diagnosis.

- CT scan and MRI scan may be arranged but these are usually normal.
- PET, SPECT and ioflupane (DaTSCAN) may measure basal ganglia dopaminergic function.

MAP 9.4 Parkinson's Disease

Treatment

- Conservative: patient education. Rehabilitation to improve gait and mobility. Regular assessment of activities of daily living.
- Medical:
  - Levodopa: crosses the blood–brain barrier (BBB) where it is converted to dopamine.
  - Carbidopa; always given with levodopa. It is a dopa decarboxylase inhibitor and prevents levodopa from being metabolised to dopamine in other regions of the body. Therefore, it acts to decrease peripheral side-effects.
  - Selegiline; inhibits monoamine oxidase B (MAO-B). This enzyme breaks down dopamine.
  - Amantadine; dopamine agonist. Decreases Parkinsonian symptoms.
  - Surgical: this option is unlikely since drug regimens have improved.

Complications

- Dysphagia.
- Dementia.
- Increased risk of falls.
- Erectile dysfunction.

What is MS?

This is thought to be a progressive autoimmune condition in which the neurons of the central nervous system demyelinate. Its progression may be classified into 4 subtypes:

1 Relapsing remitting.
2 Primary progressive.
3 Secondary progressive.
4 Benign.

Causes

The exact cause of MS is not known but there are several factors that are thought to contribute:

- It is thought to be a type IV T cell-mediated immune response.
- Location: those who live further from the equator and Sardinians are at greater risk than other populations.
- Viruses may play a role, e.g. Epstein–Barr virus (EBV).
- Smoking is a risk factor.

Pathophysiology

- Plaques of demyelination, disseminated in time and space, interfere with neuronal transmission.
- Often patients enter remission but then relapse. This is because the demyelinated neurons do not heal fully.

Signs and symptoms

- Usually monosymptomatic.
- Symptoms relate to the location where plaques of demyelination occur. Remember these as **DOTS**:
  ○ **D**iplopia, **D**ysaesthesia.
  ○ **O**ptic neuritis: this is often a presenting symptom and patients complain of double vision (diplopia).
  ○ **T**rigeminal neuralgia, **T**runk and limb ataxia.
  ○ ↓ **S**ense of vibration.
- Uhthoff's phenomenon: symptoms worsen in hot conditions.

MAP 9.5 **Multiple Sclerosis (MS)**

Treatment

- Conservative: patient education. Use diagnostic McDonald criteria and regularly assess ADLs as well as psychosocial impact of disease.
- Medical:
  ○ Interferon.
  ○ Methylprednisolone, a corticosteroid.
  ○ Glatiramer acetate, an immunomodulator.
  ○ Natalizumab, a monoclonal antibody.
  ○ Alemtuzumab, a monoclonal antibody.
  ○ Azathioprine, a purine analogue (immunosuppressant).
  ○ Mitoxantrone, a doxorubicin analogue.

Investigations

- LP: some proteins are altered in MS, e.g. oligoclonal bands.
- MRI scan: shows regions affected by inflammation and scarring, e.g. Dawson's fingers.

Complications

- Urinary incontinence.
- Bowel incontinence.
- Depression.
- Epilepsy.
- Paralysis.

MAP 9.5 Multiple Sclerosis (MS)

Musculoskeletal System

Map 10.1 Muscle Contraction

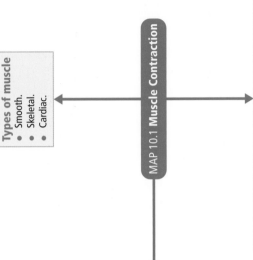

MAP 10.1 **Muscle Contraction**

Types of muscle
- Smooth.
- Skeletal.
- Cardiac.

Mechanism of skeletal and cardiac muscle contraction
- Depolarisation:
  - Action potential causes voltage gated Ca^{2+} ion channels to open.
  - Neurotransmitter released.
- Spread of depolarisation:
  - Down the T-tubules to dihydropyridine receptors in skeletal muscle.
  - In cardiac muscle, this process involves calcium-induced calcium release from the sarcoplasmic reticulum.
- Conformational change:
  - ↑ Ca^{2+} ions from calcium-induced calcium release.
  - Ca^{2+} ions bind to troponin C.
- Cross bridge formation:
  - Myosin head binds to actin when tropomyosin moves due to conformational change.
- Power stroke:
  - ADP released.
  - Muscle contracts.
- Myosin head released and cycle repeats.

Mechanism of smooth muscle contraction
- Depolarisation:
  - Caused by action potential.
  - Voltage gated Ca^{2+} ion channels open.
- Calmodulin binding: Ca^{2+} ions bind to calmodulin.
- Myosin light chain kinase (MLCK) activated.
- The role of myosin: actin coupled with myosin P causes contraction.

MAP 10.2 **Arthritis**

RHEUMATOID ARTHRITIS (RA)

What is RA?

This is a chronic, autoimmune type III hypersensitivity reaction that principally affects the joints but may also affect other organs. Joint involvement is characterised by symmetrical deformation with pain that is worse in the morning.

Cause

The exact cause of RA is unknown, but it is thought to involve a type III hypersensitivity reaction. This condition is associated with HLA DR4 and HLA DR1.

Signs and symptoms

- Hands: Z deformity, boutonnière deformity, swan neck deformity, ulnar deviation, subluxation of the fingers, Raynaud's phenomenon.
- Wrist: carpal tunnel syndrome.
- Feet: subluxation of the toes, hammer toe deformity.
- Skin: rheumatoid nodule, vasculitis.
- Cardiovascular: atherosclerosis is increased in RA.
- Respiratory: pulmonary fibrosis.
- Bones: osteoporosis.
- Pain and stiffness.

Continued overleaf

OSTEOARTHRITIS (OA)

What is OA?

This is a degenerative arthritis affecting synovial joints and is characterised by cartilage degeneration, the associated response of the periarticular tissue and pain that is typically worse at the end of the day.

Causes

Damage to the joints and general wear and tear of the joint over time is thought to be the primary cause of OA. There are certain factors that increase the risk of OA such as:

- Increased age.
- Obesity.
- Trauma to the joint.
- Conditions such as haemochromatosis and Ehlers–Danlos syndrome.

Signs and symptoms

- Pain and stiffness.
- Swelling around the joints involved.
- Crepitus.
- Heberden's nodes at distal interphalangeal (DIP) joints.
  Remember they are the 'outer Hebrides'.
- Bouchard's nodes at proximal interphalangeal (PIP) joints.

Continued overleaf

Map 10.2 Arthritis

Map 10.2 Arthritis

RA (*Continued*)

Investigations

- Bloods:
  - 80% test positive for rheumatoid factor.
  - ESR and CRP raised.
  - Cyclic citrullinated peptide (CCP) antibodies. If positive this is suggestive of erosive disease.
- Radiology: radiological signs of RA are visualised on plain film:
  - Bony erosion.
  - Subluxation.
  - Carpal instability,
  - Joint involvement of metacarpophalangeal joint (MCPJ) and metatarsophalangeal joint (MTPJ) .
  - Periarticular osteoporosis.

Treatment

- Conservative: patient education. Encourage exercise. Refer to physiotherapy and assess activities of daily living (ADLs).
- Medical: glucocorticoids, disease modifying antirheumatic drugs (DMARDs), e.g. gold salts, methotrexate, sulfasalazine. Anticytokine therapies may be considered in patients intolerant of methotrexate.
- Surgery: excision arthroplasty or replacement may be considered in severely affected joints.

Complications

- Carpal tunnel syndrome.
- Pericarditis.
- Cervical myopathy.
- Tendon rupture.
- Sjögren's syndrome.

OA (*Continued*)

Investigations

- Bloods: usually are not diagnostic but may be relevant when OA is related to another condition such as haemochromatosis.
- Radiology: radiological signs: **LOSS**
  - **L**oss of joint space.
  - **O**steophytes.
  - **S**ubchondral cysts.
  - **S**clerosis.

Treatment

- Conservative: patient education. Encourage exercise and weight loss.
- Medical:
  - Analgesia, e.g. paracetamol or nonsteroidal anti-inflammatory drugs.
  - Gels such as capsaicin may be useful.
  - Steroid injections.
- Surgical: arthroplasty.

Complications

- Increased risk of gout.
- Chondrocalcinosis.

REACTIVE ARTHRITIS

What is reactive arthritis?
This is an asymmetrical arthritis that occurs post gastrointestinal or urogenital infection.

Causes
The exact cause and pathophysiology of this condition is not known. However, it often occurs after an infection, typically, a sexually transmitted infection or an infection of the gastrointestinal tract.

Signs and symptoms
- Urethritis.
- Arthritis: pain and stiffness.
- Uveitis/conjunctivitis.

Investigations
- Bloods: seronegative for rheumatoid factor. Blood cultures. Look for infectious cause.
- Radiology: X-ray of affected joint (assesses severity).

Treatment
- Conservative: patient education. Refer to physiotherapy.
- Medical: analgesia nonsteroidal anti-inflammatory drugs (NSAIDs) and disease modifying antirheumatic drugs (DMARDs), e.g. sulphasalzine (first line).

Complications
- Arrhythmia.
- Uveitis.
- Aortic insufficiency.

Remember PEAR:
- **P**soriatic arthritis.
- **E**nteropathic arthropathies.
- **A**nkylosing spondylitis.
- **R**eactive arthritis.

MAP 10.3 **Spondyloarthropathies**

Continued overleaf

Map 10.3 Spondyloarthropathies

Musculoskeletal System

Map 10.3 Spondyloarthropathies

PSORIATIC ARTHRITIS

What is psoriatic arthritis?

This is an inflammatory arthritis that is associated with the skin condition psoriasis. It is associated with HLA B27. The signs and symptoms also depend on how and where the joints are affected. Accordingly, psoriatic arthritis may be split into 5 subtypes:

1 Asymmetrical oligoarthritis (distal and proximal interphalangeal joints).
2 Symmetrical rheumatoid-like arthropathy.
3 Ankylosing spondylitis variant.
4 Polyarteritis with skin and nail changes.
5 Arthritis mutilans.

Causes

The exact cause is unknown. It is thought to be due to an inflammatory process coupled with genetic involvement of the HLA B27 gene.
The greatest risk factor is a family history of psoriasis.

Signs and symptoms

- Psoriasis: well-demarcated salmon-pink plaques with evidence of scaling. These plaques are usually present on the extensor surfaces (chronic plaque psoriasis) but sometimes smaller plaques may occur in a raindrop pattern over the torso. This is called guttate psoriasis and is often preceded by an upper respiratory tract infection/sore throat that is caused by *Streptococcus*.
- Joint pain and stiffness.
- Swelling of affected joints.
- Nail changes: there are 4 nail changes noted in psoriasis: yellowing of the nail, onycholysis, pitting and subungual hyperkeratosis.

ENTEROPATHIC ARTHROPATHIES

What are enteropathic arthropathies?

This is an arthritis that develops in association with inflammatory bowel disease (IBD). It is indistinguishable from reactive arthritis.

Causes

The exact cause and pathophysiology of this condition are not known. However, it is thought to be associated with HLA B27.

Signs and symptoms

- Those of IBD, see page 40.
- Spondylitis.
- Sacroiliitis.
- Peripheral arthritis: usually of large joints.

Investigations

- Those for IBD, see page 40.
- Radiology: X-ray of affected joint. Assess severity.

Treatment

- Analgesia (NSAIDs).
- Treatment of IBD, see page 40.

Complications

- Severely decreased mobility with axial involvement.

MAP 10.3 **Spondyloarthropathies** (*Continued*)

ANKYLOSING SPONDYLITIS

What is ankylosing spondylitis?

This is a chronic inflammatory disease of the spine and sacroiliac joints. There is predominance in young males and the condition is associated with HLA B27 (positive in 95%).

Causes

The exact cause and pathophysiology of this condition are not known. However, it is thought to be associated with HLA B27.

Signs and symptoms

- Question mark posture.
- Bamboo spine: due to calcification of ligaments.
- Pain and stiffness: symptoms improve with exercise.

Investigations

- Bloods: seronegative for rheumatoid factor.
- Radiology: CXR and MRI scan can assess changes in the spine.

Treatment

- Conservative: patient education. Refer to physiotherapy.
- Medical: analgesia (NSAIDs) and DMARDs, e.g. sulphasalzine (first line).
- Surgery: corrective spinal surgery.

Complications

- Osteoprosis.
- Spinal fractures.
- Increased risk of cardiovascular disease, e.g. stroke and myocardial infarction.

Investigations

- Psoriasis is a clinical diagnosis.
- Bloods: seronegative for rheumatoid factor.
- Radiology: 'Pencil-in-cup' deformity on hand X-ray. X-ray of affected joints to assess severity.

Treatment

- Conservative: patient education. Refer to physiotherapy. Explain to patients that psoriasis does not have a cure and control of the disease is more realistic.
- Medical: analgesia (nonsteroidal anti-inflammatory drugs [NSAIDs]) and disease modifying antirheumatic drugs (DMARDs), e.g. methotrexate (first line). Manage psoriasis.
- Surgery: rarely joint replacement.

Complications

- Neurological manifestations if atlanto–axial joint involvement.
- Joint destruction.

Map 10.3 Spondyloarthropathies

Map 10.4 Gout

What is gout?

Gout is an inflammatory crystal monoarthropathy caused by the deposition of urate crystals.

These monosodium urate crystals often precipitate in the metatarsophalangeal joint (MTPJ).

Gout involving the big toe is known as a podagra.

Causes

There are many causes of gout but essentially anything that increases urate levels may be the underlying cause. Some examples include,

Horrific **DELAY:**

- **H**yperuricaemia, **H**ereditary.
- **D**iuretics (thiazides).
- **E**thanol.
- **L**eukaemia.
- ren**A**l impairment.
- associated with Lesch–N**Y**han syndrome.

Signs and symptoms

- Calor, dolor, rubor and tumour (heat, pain, redness and swelling) of the affected joint, which is usually the MTPJ in 50% of patients.
- Tophi (urate deposits) may be present on tendon surfaces, e.g. the elbow, or visible on the ear.
- Patients may have symptoms of renal calculi.

Investigations

- Bloods: serum urate levels, FBC, WCC, U&Es, creatinine, ESR, CRP.
- GFR: assess kidney function.
- Synovial fluid analysis: positive if birefringent monosodium urate crystals seen.

MAP 10.4 **Gout**

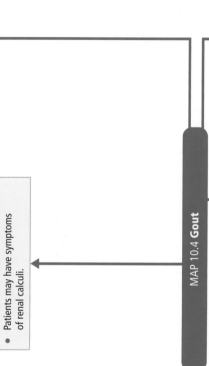

Pseudogout vs. gout

Characteristic	Pseudogout	Gout
Joints affected	Larger proximal	Classically 1st MTPJ
Crystal type	Calcium pyrophosphate crystals	Sodium urate crystals
Crystal shape	Rhomboid	Needle
Light microscopy	Negative birefringence	Strongly positive birefringence

Treatment

- Conservative: patient education. Lifestyle advice, e.g. encourage alcohol reduction and a low purine diet. Review medications that the patient is taking and stop causative agents, e.g. thiazide diuretics, if possible.
- Medical:
  - Analgesia.
  - Acute: colchicine and steroids.
  - Chronic: allopurinol. Febuxostat may be used if allopurinol is not tolerated by the patient.

Complications

- Joint damage.
- Renal calculi.
- Tophi formation.

Map 10.4 Gout

Map 10.5 Bone Tumours

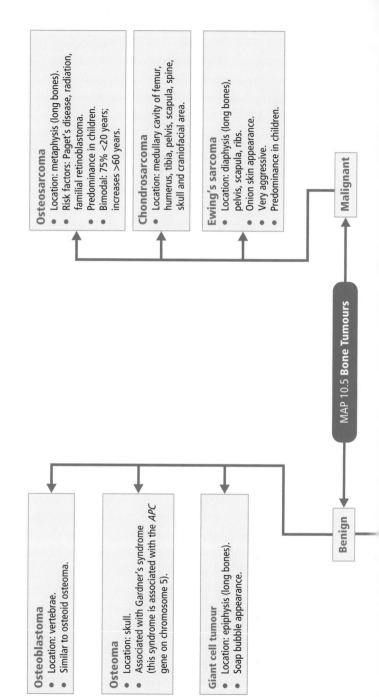

Osteoblastoma
- Location: vertebrae.
- Similar to osteoid osteoma.

Osteoma
- Location: skull.
- Associated with Gardner's syndrome (this syndrome is associated with the *APC* gene on chromosome 5).

Giant cell tumour
- Location: epiphysis (long bones).
- Soap bubble appearance.

Benign

MAP 10.5 **Bone Tumours**

Malignant

Osteosarcoma
- Location: metaphysis (long bones).
- Risk factors: Paget's disease, radiation, familial retinoblastoma.
- Predominance in children.
- Bimodal: 75% <20 years; increases >60 years.

Chondrosarcoma
- Location: medullary cavity of femur, humerus, tibia, pelvis, scapula, spine, skull and craniofacial area.

Ewing's sarcoma
- Location: diaphysis (long bones), pelvis, scapula, ribs.
- Onion skin appearance.
- Very aggressive.
- Predominance in children.

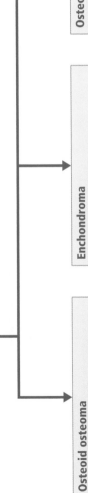

Osteoid osteoma
- Location: femur and tibia, phalanges and vertebrae.
- Intracortical lesion best differentiated on CT.
- Nidus.

Enchondroma
- Location: intramedullary bone.
- Cartilaginous neoplasm.
- Seen in phalanges.

Osteochondroma
- Location: metaphysis (long bones).
- Most common benign bone lesion.

Map 10.5 Bone Tumours

Map 10.6 Metabolic Bone Disease

MAP 10.6 **Metabolic Bone Disease**

OSTEOPOROSIS

What is osteoporosis?

This is a bone disorder that is characterised by loss of trabecular bone and increased fracture risk. It is more common in postmenopausal women due to ↓ oestrogen levels and ↑ bone resorption.

Causes

There is no single cause of osteoporosis but there are risk factors that predispose patients to this condition. These include:

- Loss of protective oestrogen in postmenopausal women.
- Prolonged steroid use.
- Increasing age.
- Excessive alcohol intake.
- Smoking.
- Positive family history.
- Diet deficient in calcium.
- Endocrine disorders such as diabetes mellitus and hyperthyroidism.

Signs and symptoms

This is often asymptomatic until the patient presents with pathological fracture. Patients may report loss in height, back pain and have a dowager's hump (hyperkyphosis) on physical examination.

OSTEOMALACIA

What is osteomalacia?

This is a metabolic bone disorder characterised by low mineral bone content and deficient vitamin D. This leads to soft bones; however, the amount of bone is normal. In children this condition is called rickets.

Causes

Remember **REVOLT:**

- **RE**sistance to vitamin D.
- **V**itamin D deficiency.
- **O**steodystrophy (renal).
- **L**iver disease.
- **T**umour-induced osteomalacia.

Signs and symptoms

- Bone pain.
- Myalgia.
- Pathological fracture.

Investigations

- Bloods: FBC, U&Es, LFTs, TFTs, glucose, serum calcium, serum phosphate, alkaline phosphatase, PTH and vitamin D levels.
- Radiology: X-ray to assess fractures.

Investigations

- Bloods: FBC, U&Es, LFTs, TFTs, glucose, serum calcium, serum phosphate, alkaline phosphatase levels and PTH.
- Dual-energy X-ray (DEXA) scan: a T-score >−2.5 is diagnostic.
- Radiology: X-ray, CT and MRI scan to assess fractures.

Treatment

- Conservative: patient education. Modify risk factors, e.g. smoking and alcohol cessation. Encourage weight-bearing exercise. Assess activities of daily living.
- Medical: selective oestrogen receptor modulators (SERMs), calcitonin and bisphosphonates.

Treatment

- Conservative: patient education. Dietary advice concerning calcium and vitamin D intake.
- Medical: vitamin D supplements, e.g. cholecalciferol and calcitriol.

Complications

- Increased risk of fracture.

Map continues overleaf

Map 10.6 Metabolic Bone Disease

MAP 10.6 **Metabolic Bone Disease** (*Continued*)

Map 10.6 Metabolic Bone Disease

OSTEOPETROSIS
What is osteopetrosis?
This condition, also known as marble bone disease, occurs when osteoclasts do not function properly. As such bone is no longer resorbed. This means that bones are thick and fracture easily.

Causes
- Osteoclast dysfunction.

Signs and symptoms
- Asymptomatic.
- Hepatomegaly.
- Splenomegaly.
- Anaemia.

Investigations
- Bloods: FBC, U&Es, LFTs, TFTs, glucose, serum calcium, serum phosphate, alkaline phosphatase and PTH.
- Radiology: X-ray to assess fractures.

Treatment
- Conservative: patient education. Refer to physiotherapy.
- Medical: vitamin D, calcitriol, erythropoietin, corticosteroids, gamma interferon, bone marrow transplant.

Complications
- Increased fracture risk.
- Neurological involvement due to nerve impingement.

PAGET'S DISEASE
What is Paget's disease?
This is a chronic remodelling disorder of bone that results in abnormal bone architecture.

Causes
The exact cause is unknown but it this thought to have a viral and genetic aetiology.

Signs and symptoms
- Asymptomatic.
- Bone pain.
- Pathological fracture.
- Hearing loss (if skull affected).

Investigations
- Bloods: FBC, U&Es, LFTs, TFTs, glucose, serum calcium, serum phosphate, alkaline phosphatase and PTH.
- Radiology: X-ray to assess fractures.

Treatment
- Conservative: patient education and management of complications.
- Medical: bisphosphonates such as zoledronate injections.

Complications
- Osteogenic sarcoma.
- Heart failure.
- Increased risk of renal calculi.

TABLE 10.1 Biochemical Profiling in Different Metabolic Bone Diseases

Investigation	Osteoporosis	Osteomalacia	Osteopetrosis	Paget's disease
Serum calcium	Normal	↓	Normal	Normal
Serum phosphate	Normal	↓	Normal	Normal
Alkaline phosphatase	Normal	↑	↑	Varies with evolution of disease
PTH	Normal	↑	Normal	Normal

Table 10.1 Biochemical Profiling in Different Metabolic Bone Diseases

TABLE 10.2 **Brachial Plexus Injury**

Nerve and nerve origin	Lesion	Cause	Comment
Axillary nerve (C5–C6)	Deltoid muscle paralysis	Shoulder dislocation Humeral neck fracture	Atrophy of the deltoid muscle seen
Musculocutaneous nerve (C5–C7)	Paralysis of biceps, brachialis and coracobrachialis muscles	Rarely occurs Complication of surgery Dislocation	↓ Sensation of lateral forearm
Median nerve (C5–T1)	Above antecubital fossa	Supracondylar fractures Neuropathy	Papal sign of benediction Ape hand deformity (at rest) Loss of sensation over thenar eminence
	Below antecubital fossa	Injury to the anterior interosseous branch of the median nerve	Anterior interosseous syndrome Inability to pronate the forearm
	At the wrist	Laceration of the wrist	Papal sign of benediction Ape hand deformity (at rest) Loss of sensation over thenar eminence
	Within the wrist	Carpal tunnel syndrome (CTS)	Parasthesiae in median nerve distribution, i.e. lateral 2.5 fingers Pain often worse at night Wasting seen over the thenar eminence Special tests may be used in the diagnosis of CTS: Phalen's test and Tinel's test CTS is associated with pregnancy, the oral contraceptive pill, diabetes, heart failure, acromegaly, rheumatoid arthritis and gout

Table 10.2 Brachial Plexus Injury

Ulnar nerve (C8–T1)	Ulnar clawing	Cubital tunnel syndrome Ganglion cyst in the Guyon canal	Ulnar clawing is more pronounced the more distal the lesion. This is known as the ulnar paradox.
Radial nerve (C5–C8)	Wrist drop	Trauma: fracture of the humerus Lead poisoning	If lesion is located at the axilla it is sometimes called Saturday night palsy
C5 and C6 roots	Erb–Duchenne palsy, aka waiter's tip palsy	Dystocia (difficult childbirth)	Paralysis of lateral rotators: infraspinatus, teres minor Paralysis of abductors: supraspinatus, deltoid Paralysis of supinators: biceps Paralysis of flexors: brachialis
C8 and T1	Klumpke's palsy	Dystocia	Atrophy of interosseous muscles Atrophy of thenar muscles Atrophy of hypothenar muscles ↓ Sensation of medial hand and medial forearm

Table 10.2 Brachial Plexus Injury

Map 11.1 Reproductive Hormones

OESTROGEN
Secreted by
- Ovaries and placenta.

Function
- Genital development.
- Breast development.
- Follicle growth.
- Endometrial growth.
- Upregulates oestrogen, LH and progesterone receptors.
- Inhibits FSH and LH through feedback mechanism.
- Stimulates prolactin secretion.
- Stimulates LH surge, which causes ovulation.
- Increases protein transport.

INHIBIN
Secreted by
- Sertoli cells.

Function
- Inhibits FSH.

PROGESTERONE
Secreted by
- Corpus luteum, placenta, adrenal cortex and testes.

Function
- Maintains pregnancy.
- Produces cervical mucus.
- Increases body temperature.
- Inhibits LH and FSH.
- Relaxes uterine smooth muscle.
- Downregulates oestrogen receptors.
- Increases endometrial gland secretion.
- Increases spiral artery development.
- Softens ligaments during pregnancy.

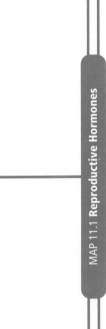

MAP 11.1 **Reproductive Hormones**

FOLLICLE STIMULATING HORMONE (FSH)

Secreted by
- Anterior pituitary gland.

Function
- Stimulates Sertoli cells to produce androgen binding protein.
- Stimulates Sertoli cells to produce inhibin.

TESTOSTERONE

Secreted by
- Leydig cells of the testes and adrenal cortex.

Function
- Male secondary sexual characteristics.
- Penile and muscular development.
- Growth of seminal vesicles.
- Epiphyseal plate closure.
- Differentiation of vas deferens, seminal vesicles and epididymis.

LUTEINISING HORMONE (LH)

Secreted by
- Anterior pituitary gland.

Function
- Stimulates Leydig cells to produce testosterone.
- Surge causes ovulation.

Map 11.1 Reproductive Hormones

Figure 11.1 The Menstrual Cycle

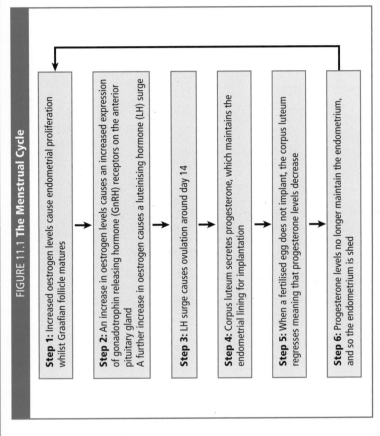

FIGURE 11.1 The Menstrual Cycle

Step 1: Increased oestrogen levels cause endometrial proliferation whilst Graafian follicle matures

Step 2: An increase in oestrogen levels causes an increased expression of gonadotrophin releasing hormone (GnRH) receptors on the anterior pituitary gland
A further increase in oestrogen causes a luteinising hormone (LH) surge

Step 3: LH surge causes ovulation around day 14

Step 4: Corpus luteum secretes progesterone, which maintains the endometrial lining for implantation

Step 5: When a fertilised egg does not implant, the corpus luteum regresses meaning that progesterone levels decrease

Step 6: Progesterone levels no longer maintain the endometrium, and so the endometrium is shed

FIGURE 11.2 **The Lactation Pathway**

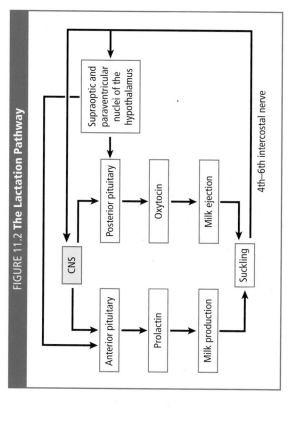

Map 11.2 Pregnancy and Lactation

MATERNAL CHANGES DURING PREGNANCY

Respiratory system
- Elevated diaphragm by 4 cm.
- ↓ Expiratory reserve volume.
- ↑ Tidal volume.

Cardiovascular system
- ↓ BP because progesterone decreases vascular resistance by increasing spiral artery formation.
- ↑ Cardiac output.
- ↑ Blood volume since renin angiotensin aldosterone system (RAAS) is stimulated by lowered BP.
- Constriction of peripheral circulation (this is why some pregnant women experience Raynaud's phenomenon).

Renal system
- ↑ Kidney size.
- ↑ Frequency of urination.
- ↑ Glomerular filtration rate (GFR).
- ↑ Urinary tract infection risk due to dilated, elongated ureters.

Musculoskeletal system
- Gait changes.
- Lower back pain.
- Ligaments soften.
- Symphysis pubis dysfunction.

MASTITIS

What is mastitis?
This is inflammation of the breast tissue.

Causes
Milk stasis or overproduction causes regional infection of the breast parenchyma with *Staphylococcus aureus*, which enters the breast via trauma to the nipple. This in turn causes mastitis.

Signs and symptoms
- Calor, dolor, rubor and tumour (heat, pain, redness and swelling) of the breast tissue.
- Nipple discharge.
- Fever.

Investigations
- This is a clinical diagnosis.

Treatment
- Conservative: patient education. Encourage mother to continue breastfeeding since this will help to overcome the obstruction.
- Medical: flucloxacillin.

Dermatology
- Linea nigra.
- Palmar erythema.
- Spider angioma.

Gastrointestinal system
- Constipation.
- Gastro-oesophageal reflux disease.
- ↑ Risk of gallstones.
- Gestational diabetes.

Reproductive system
- ↑ Uterus size.
- Thickening of uterine ligaments.
- Softening of cervix.
- ↑ Vaginal secretions.

Immune system
- Weakened.

MAP 11.2 **Pregnancy and Lactation**

Map 11.2 Pregnancy and Lactation

TABLE 11.1 **Breast Tumours**

Breast tumour	Benign or malignant	Characteristics	Investigations	Treatment	Complications
Fibroadenoma	Benign	Small Also known as 'breast mouse' due to tumour not being tethered Sharp edges Most common type of benign breast tumour in young women	Undergo triple assessment: 1 Examination 2 Imaging 3 Biopsy Physical examination for lumps and masses Bloods: FBC, WCC, U&Es, LFTs, TFTs Radiology: mammogram, ultrasound scan, fine needle biopsy under ultrasound guidance (core needle biopsy may be required). Look for metastasis with CXR, CT scan and MRI scan Risk factors for breast cancer: • Female • Increasing age • Family history of breast cancer	Treatment depends on the cause of the breast tumour and whether it is benign or malignant; treatment may be split into 3 modalities: 1 Conservative: patient and family education; refer to Macmillan nurses; offer genetic counselling; provide psychological assessment and support 2 Medical: prognosis of disease is assessed using the Nottingham Prognostic Index (NPI): $NPI = (0.2 \times invasive\ size) + lymph\ node\ stage + grade\ of\ tumour$ Medical therapy may be split into adjuvant hormone therapy, chemotherapy or	Death Metastasis Complications of chemotherapy regimen Complications of radiotherapy regimen Depression
Intraductal papilloma	Benign	Small Under areola Bloody discharge from nipple			
Phyllodes tumour	Benign	Large Leaf-like projections Rapid growing			
Ductal carcinoma in situ (DCIS)	Malignant	From ductal hyperplasia Cheesy discharge, confined to ducts			
Comedocarcinoma	Malignant	High-grade DCIS Characterised by central necrosis Cheesy discharge			

Table 11.1 Breast Tumours

Invasive ductal	Malignant	A hard mass
		Sharp edges
		Most common
		Very aggressive
			• Genetic involvement, e.g. BRCA 1 (chromosome 17) and BRCA 2 (chromosome 13)
			• Alcohol
			• Obesity
			• Increased oestrogen exposure, e.g.:
			  ○ Early menarche
			  ○ Late menopause
			  ○ Oral contraceptive pill use
			  ○ Hormone replacement therapy
			  ○ Decreased parity
			  ○ Not breastfeeding
				HER2 directed therapy, depending on the type of tumour
				Hormone treatment: premenopausal women are treated with tamoxifen (a selective oestrogen receptor modulator); postmenopausal women are treated with anastrazole (an aromatase inhibitor). This is because trials such as the ATAC trial have suggested that aromatase inhibitors are superior to tamoxifen in postmenopausal women. If a woman becomes menopausal during treatment she will benefit from switching medications
				Chemotherapy and radiotherapy regimens: vary depending on tumour type

Invasive lobular	Malignant	Bilateral presentation		
Medullary	Malignant	Well differentiated Lacks desmoplastic reaction Lymphatic infiltrate Good prognosis		
Inflammatory	Malignant	Invades the dermis and lymphatic system Peau d'orange appearance Retracted nipple		
Paget's disease of the breast	Malignant	Epidermal infiltration of ductal carcinoma Eczematoid nipple changes		

Continued overleaf

Table 11.1 Breast Tumours

TABLE 11.1 **Breast Tumours** (*Continued*)

Breast tumour	Benign or malignant	Characteristics	Investigations	Treatment	Complications
				HER2 directed therapy: treatment with trastuzumab (herceptin). This is a monoclonal antibody against the extracellular domain of the HER2 receptor 3 Surgical: the primary aim of surgery is to remove the invasive and noninvasive cancer with clear margins. Lumpectomy followed by a radiotherapy regime has been shown to be as effective as mastectomy, but mastectomy may be recommended in certain circumstances such as multifocal breast disease. The ipsilateral axilla should also be assessed with ultrasound, fine needle aspiration or core biopsy.	

Table 11.1 Breast Tumours

					Clinical staging of the axilla should also be assessed by sentinel lymph node biopsy. The reason for this is to avoid unnecessary axillary clearance in patients

Table 11.1 Breast Tumours

The Reproductive System

What is BPH?

This is a benign enlargement of the prostate gland, particularly in the transitional zone. It is common with increasing age.

Causes

There is hypertrophy of the epithelial and stromal cells of the prostate gland. This classically occurs in the transitional zone of the prostate gland and is thought to be driven by the androgen dihydrotestosterone.

Signs and symptoms

Remember **FUN BOO**:

- **F**requency.
- **U**rgency.
- **N**octuria.
- Those of bladder outflow obstruction (**BOO**):
  - **H**esitancy.
  - **I**ntermittent flow/poor urine stream/dribbling.
  - **I**ncomplete bladder emptying.

Investigations

- Per rectum (PR) examination: an enlarged but smooth prostate gland with a palpable midline sulcus.
- Urine dipstick, microscopy and culture.
- Bloods: FBCs, U&Es and creatinine (renal function), LFTs.
- Prostate specific antigen (PSA) – usually raised.
- Radiology: ultrasound scan of the urinary tract, transrectal ultrasound scan.

Management

- Conservative: watchful waiting is usually adopted in mild disease.
- Completion of the International Prostate Symptom Score (IPSS). Completion of a voiding diary to see if patient is bothered by their symptoms.
- Medical:
  - α1-adrenoreceptor blockers, e.g. tamsulosin.
  - 5α-reductase inhibitors, e.g. finasteride.
- Surgical:
  - Transurethral resection of the prostate (TURP).

Complications

- Urinary retention.
- Recurrent urinary tract infections.
- Impaired renal function.
- Haematuria.

MAP 11.3 **Benign Prostatic Hyperplasia (BPH)**

FIGURE 11.3 **Zones of the Prostate Gland**

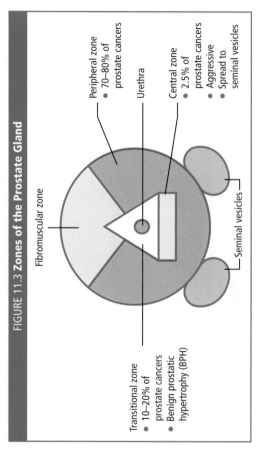

Peripheral zone
• 70–80% of prostate cancers

Urethra

Central zone
• 2.5% of prostate cancers
• Aggressive
• Spread to seminal vesicles

Fibromuscular zone

Transitional zone
• 10–20% of prostate cancers
• Benign prostatic hypertrophy (BPH)

Seminal vesicles

Figure 11.3 Zones of the Prostate Gland

Map 11.4 Prostate Cancer

MAP 11.4 Prostate Cancer

Investigations

- Per rectum (PR) examination: an enlarged prostate gland that may be uninodular or multinodular. The midline sulcus is usually no longer palpable.
- Urine dipstick, microscopy and culture.
- Bloods: FBCs, U&Es and creatinine (renal function), LFTs.
- Prostate specific antigen (PSA) – usually raised.
- Radiology: transrectal ultrasound and biopsy. If this procedure diagnoses a malignancy then the patient should be sent for a MRI and bone scan to look for distant metastases. Prostate cancer is staged using the TMN system. Since there may also be symptoms of BOO an ultrasound scan of the urinary tract may also be required.

Management

- Conservative: involvement of Macmillan nurses and psychological support.
- Medical:
  - Radiotherapy.
  - Brachytherapy.
  - Goserelin (Zoladex) – a luteinising hormone-releasing hormone (LHRH) agonist.
  - Antiandrogens, e.g. cyproterone.
- Surgical:
  - Laparoscopic radical prostatectomy.
  - Transurethral resection of the prostate (TURP).

Complications

- Metastasis.
- Death.
- Urinary incontinence.
- Erectile dysfunction.

What is prostate cancer?

This is usually an adenocarcinoma that arises from the peripheral zone of the prostate gland.

Risk factors

- Increasing age.
- Family history of prostate cancer.
- More common in African populations.

Signs and symptoms

- Those of benign prostatic hyperplasia – FUN BOO (see page 184).
- Those of metastatic disease:
  - Weight loss.
  - Malaise and fatigue.
  - Usually spreads to bone, therefore bone pain, pathological fracture.

Map 12.1 Fertilisation

MAP 12.1 **Fertilisation**

The germ layers and their derivatives
- Ectoderm → epidermis, nervous system.
- Mesoderm → muscles, bones connective tissue.
- Endoderm → other organs, e.g. GIT, respiratory tract.

Important dates to remember
- Day 6: implantation.
- Day 9:
  ○ Blastocyst embedded in the endometrium.
  ○ Lacunae formation.
- Day 15: gastrulation.

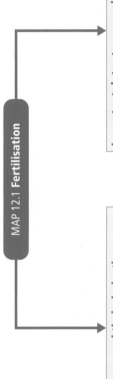

FIGURE 12.1 Development of the Embryo

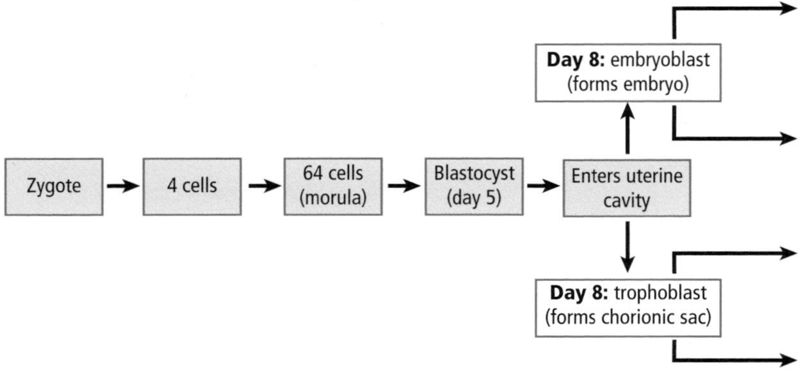

Hypoblast
- Exocoelomic membrane (Heuser's membrane)
- The hypoblast and exocoelomic membrane form the yolk sac

Epiblast
- The small cavity within the epiblast is the amniotic cavity which fills with amniotic fluid
- Amniotic fluid acts as a shock absorber and serves to regulate fetal temperature

Syncytiotrophoblast
- No distinct cell boundaries
- Creates enzymes during implantation

Cytotrophoblast
- Distinct cell boundaries
- Between embryoblast and syncytiotrophoblast

Zygote → 4 cells → 64 cells (morula) → Blastocyst (day 5) → Enters uterine cavity

Day 8: embryoblast (forms embryo)

Day 8: trophoblast (forms chorionic sac)

Figure 12.1 Development of the Embryo

Map 12.2 The Heart

Development of the heart

- Develops during week 3 from cardiac progenitor cells.
- The heart tube forms from 2 endocardial tubes at day 21 and the heart begins to beat on day 22. Note that blood flows through the endocardial tube caudocranially:
  - Truncus arteriosus → aorta and pulmonary trunk.
  - Bulbus cordis → smooth part of right ventricle (conus arteriosus); smooth part of left ventricle (aortic vestibule).
  - Primitive ventricle → Trabeculated part of right and left ventricle.
  - Primitive atrium → Trabeculated part of right and left atrium.
  - Sinus venosus → Smooth part of right atrium; coronary sinus; oblique vein of left atrium.
- The ventricle grows at a faster rate than the other areas causing the cardiac loop to fold in a U shape.
- The cardiac septa form between the 27th and 37th day.

Cardiovascular teratogens

Remember **RAT**:

- **R**etinoic acid, **R**ubella virus.
- **A**lcohol.
- **T**halidomide.

MAP 12.2 The Heart

Molecular regulation

- NKX-2.5: induces heart formation and also plays a role in expression of *HAND 1* and *HAND2*, which are important regulators of ventricle differentiation. WNT inhibitors.
- BMP2 and BMP4 along with WNT inhibitors are responsible for NKX-2.5 expression.
- Laterality-inducing genes *NODAL* and *LEFTY2* cause PITX2 expression: plays a role in cardiac loop formation.

Examples of defects

- Atrial septal defect (ASD): ostium secundum defect.
- Ostium primum defect.
- Tricuspid atresia.
- Ebstein's anomaly.
- Ventricular septal defect (VSD).
- Tetralogy of Fallot (TOF):
  - Pulmonary stenosis.
  - Overriding aorta.
  - VSD.
  - Right ventricular hypertrophy.
- Transposition of the great vessels.
- Persistent truncus arteriosus.

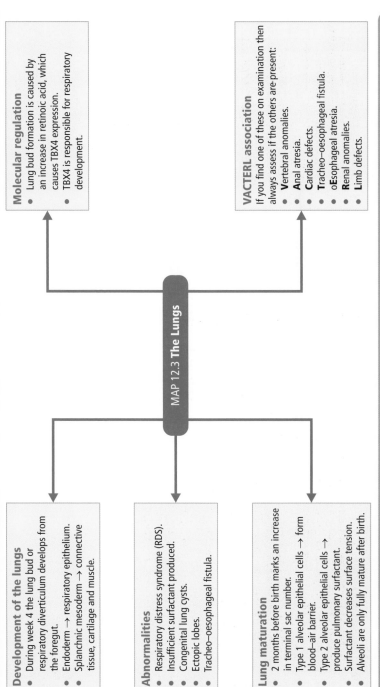

Molecular regulation
- Lung bud formation is caused by an increase in retinoic acid, which causes TBX4 expression.
- TBX4 is responsible for respiratory development.

VACTERL association
If you find one of these on examination then always assess if the others are present:
- **V**ertebral anomalies.
- **A**nal atresia.
- **C**ardiac defects.
- **T**racheo–oesophageal fistula.
- o**E**sophageal atresia.
- **R**enal anomalies.
- **L**imb defects.

MAP 12.3 **The Lungs**

Development of the lungs
- During week 4 the lung bud or respiratory diverticulum develops from the foregut.
- Endoderm → respiratory epithelium.
- Splanchnic mesoderm → connective tissue, cartilage and muscle.

Abnormalities
- Respiratory distress syndrome (RDS).
- Insufficient surfactant produced.
- Congenital lung cysts.
- Ectopic lobes.
- Tracheo–oesophageal fistula.

Lung maturation
- 2 months before birth marks an increase in terminal sac number.
- Type 1 alveolar epithelial cells → form blood–air barrier.
- Type 2 alveolar epithelial cells → produce pulmonary surfactant.
- Surfactant decreases surface tension.
- Alveoli are only fully mature after birth.

Embryology

Map 12.3 The Lungs

Map 12.4 The Gastrointestinal Tract (GIT)

Development of the GIT

There are 4 parts to the primitive gut. These are the:

1 Pharyngeal gut.
2 Foregut.
3 Midgut.
4 Hindgut.

- Endoderm → epithelial lining, pancreatic endocrine glands, pancreatic exocrine glands and hepatocytes.
- Visceral mesoderm → connective tissue and muscle.

MAP 12.4
The Gastrointestinal Tract (GIT)

Molecular regulation

Region of GIT	Gene involved
Oesophagus	SOX-2
Stomach	SOX-2
Small intestine	CDXC HOX 9, 10
Caecum	HOX 9–11
Large intestine	CDXA HOX 9–12
Cloaca	HOX 9–13
Rectum	CDXA
Liver	HOX
Duodenum	PDX1

Sonic hedgehog (SHH) gene causes epithelial–mesenchymal interaction and HOX gene expression.

Abnormalities

- Oesophageal atresia.
- Congenital hiatus hernia.
- Pyloric stenosis.
- Accessory hepatic ducts.
- Duplication of gallbladder.
- Extrahepatic biliary atresia.
- Annular pancreas.
- Omphalocoele.
- Gastroschisis.
- Rectourethral fistula.
- Rectovaginal fistula.
- Hirschsprung's disease.

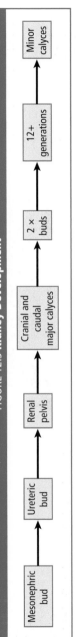

MAP 12.5 **The Kidneys**

Development of the kidneys

3 sets of kidneys form during development:

1 Pronephros: nonfunctional.
2 Mesonephros: semi-functional.
3 Metanephros: permanent kidneys.

The kidneys develop from intermediate mesoderm.

Abnormalities

● Autosomal recessive polycystic kidney disease (ARPKD).
● Autosomal dominant polycystic kidney disease (ADPKD).
● Wilms' tumour.
● Denys–Drash syndrome.
● Renal agenesis.
● Pelvic kidney.
● Horseshoe kidney.

FIGURE 12.2 **Molecular Regulation of Kidney Development**

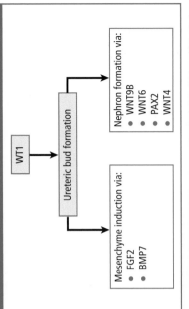

Ureteric bud formation

WT1

Mesenchyme induction via:
● FGF2
● BMP7

Nephron formation via:
● WNT9B
● WNT6
● PAX2
● WNT4

FIGURE 12.3 **Kidney Development**

Mesonephric bud → Ureteric bud → Renal pelvis → Cranial and caudal major calyces → 2 × buds → 12+ generations → Minor calyces

Map 12.5 The Kidneys

Figure 12.4 Brain Development

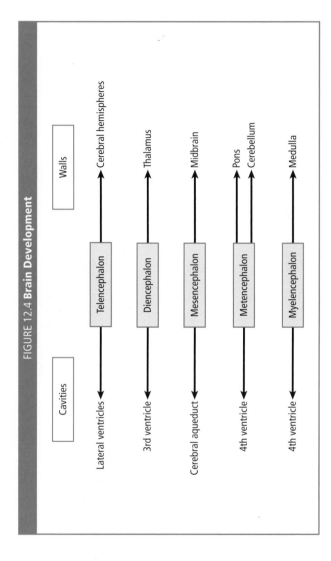

FIGURE 12.4 **Brain Development**

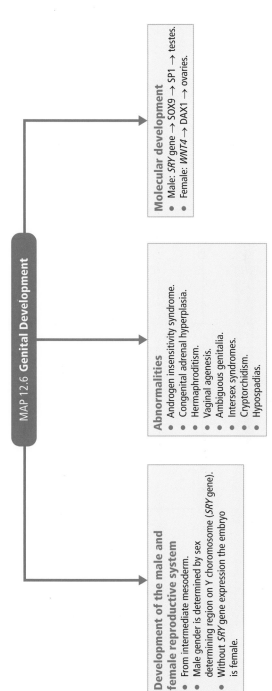

MAP 12.6 **Genital Development**

Development of the male and female reproductive system
- From intermediate mesoderm.
- Male gender is determined by sex determining region on Y choromosome (*SRY* gene).
- Without *SRY* gene expression the embryo is female.

Abnormalities
- Androgen insensitivity syndrome.
- Congenital adrenal hyperplasia.
- Hermaphroditism.
- Vaginal agenesis.
- Ambiguous genitalia.
- Intersex syndromes.
- Cryptorchidism.
- Hypospadias.

Molecular development
- Male: *SRY* gene → SOX9 → SP1 → testes.
- Female: *WNT4* → DAX1 → ovaries.

Map 12.6 Genital Development

Figure 12.5 Development of the Reproductive System

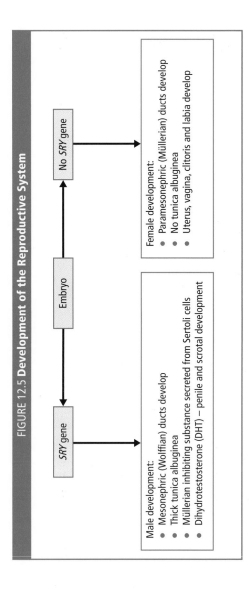

FIGURE 12.5 **Development of the Reproductive System**

Male development:
- Mesonephric (Wolffian) ducts develop
- Thick tunica albuginea
- Müllerian inhibiting substance secreted from Sertoli cells
- Dihydrotestosterone (DHT) – penile and scrotal development

Female development:
- Paramesonephric (Müllerian) ducts develop
- No tunica albuginea
- Uterus, vagina, clitoris and labia develop

SRY gene

Embryo

No *SRY* gene

Chapter Thirteen **Genetic Disorders**

HAEMOPHILIA A

What is haemophilia A?

This is an X-linked recessive bleeding and bruising disorder.

Causes

- Deficiency of factor VIII.

Signs and symptoms

These vary depending on disease severity. Bleeding is the main feature and this is prolonged, resulting in the need for investigations to uncover the cause. Positive family history may tailor diagnosis.

Investigations

- Low factor VIII levels: the lower the level, the more severe the disease.
- Coagulation factor assay.
- Increased PTT but normal PT.

Treatment

- Conservative: patient and parent education. Genetic counselling and testing is now available. Avoid anticoagulant medication, e.g. nonsteroidal anti-inflammatory drugs (NSAIDs), warfarin, aspirin.
- Medical:
  - Mild: desmopressin.
  - Severe: require IV replacement with plasma concentrate factor VIII.

Complications

- Patient's immune system may start to reject the IV plasma concentrate factor VIII by making inhibitors.
- Joint destruction by recurrent bleeding.

MAP 13.1 **X-linked Recessive Disorders**

HAEMOPHILIA B
What is haemophilia B?
Haemophilia B, also known as Christmas disease, is an X-linked recessive bleeding and bruising disorder.

Causes
- Deficiency of factor IX.

Signs and symptoms
These vary depending on disease severity. Bleeding is the main feature of this disease and this is prolonged, resulting in the need for tests to uncover the cause. Positive family history may tailor diagnosis.

Investigations
- Low factor IX levels: the lower the level, the more severe the disease.
- Coagulation factor assay.
- Increased PTT but normal PT.

Treatment
- Conservative: patient and parent education. Genetic counselling and testing is now available. Avoid anticoagulant medication, e.g. NSAIDs, warfarin, aspirin.
- Medical: IV infusion of factor IX.

Complications
- Joint destruction by recurrent bleeding.

Map 13.1 X-linked Recessive Disorders

Map 13.2 X-linked Recessive Disorders

DUCHENNE MUSCULAR DYSTROPHY

What is Duchenne muscular dystrophy?

This is a form of muscular dystrophy.

Causes

- Mutated dystrophin gene at locus Xp21.

Signs and symptoms

- Patient falls frequently.
- Fatigue.
- Toe walking/difficulty walking.
- Muscle weakness.
- Muscle pseudohypertrophy.
- Muscle fibrosis.
- Positive Gower's test.

Investigations

- DNA testing: confirms mutation of dystrophin gene.
- Creatine phosphokinase test. Results show increased levels.
- Muscle biopsy: confirms mutation of dystrophin gene.
- Electromyography (EMG): analyses muscle destruction.

Treatment

There is no specific treatment for this disease. Prednisolone and creatinine replacement may be considered. Patient will be wheelchair bound at ~12 years; refer to occupational therapy and physiotherapy. Patient and parent education and support is essential since this condition is very debilitating and life expectancy is ~25–30 years.

Complications

- Scoliosis.
- Respiratory complications and increased risk of respiratory infections.
- Cardiomyopathy.
- Osteoporosis.

MAP 13.2 **X-linked Recessive Disorders** (*Continued*)

LESCH–NYHAN SYNDROME

What is Lesch–Nyhan syndrome?

This is a rare X-linked recessive disorder that causes a build-up of uric acid in the body.

Causes

- Deficiency of hypoxanthine–guanine phosphoribosyltransferase (HGPRT).

Signs and symptoms

- Behavioural problems.
- Intellectual impairment.
- Self-harming behaviour.
- Poor muscle control.
- Symptoms of gout, see page 162.

Investigations

- Bloods: FBC, U&Es, LFTs, creatinine, uric acid, HGPRT.
- Radiology: ultrasound scan of kidneys for radiolucent urate renal calculi.

Treatment

- Conservative: parent education.
- Medical: allopurinol (to decrease uric acid levels). For neurological and behavioural problems consider benzodiazepines and baclofen.

Complications

- Gout.
- Renal calculi.
- Self harm.

Map 13.2 X-linked Recessive Disorders

RETT'S SYNDROME

What is Rett's syndrome?

This is a neurodevelopmental disorder of brain grey matter.

Causes

- Mutation of the methyl-CpG binding protein-2 (*MECP2*) gene.

Signs and symptoms

- Neurological dysfunction, e.g.:
  - Ataxia.
  - Hypotonia.
  - Inability to walk or altered gait.
  - Chorea.
- Autistic behaviour, e.g.:
  - Lack of eye contact.
  - Lack of theory of mind.
  - Decreased social interaction.
  - Speech deficit.
  - Screaming.

Investigations

- DNA sequencing of *MECP2* gene is diagnostic.

Treatment

- Conservative: parent education.
- Medical: treatment of complications.

AICARDI SYNDROME

What is Aicardi syndrome?

This is an X-linked recessive condition in which there is partial or a complete absence of the corpus callosum. Retinal abnormalities and seizures are also present.

Causes

The exact cause remains unknown but it is thought to be due to new mutations that are passed genetically to offspring via X-linked recessive inheritance.

Signs and symptoms

- Infantile spasms.

Investigations

- Radiology: CT or MRI scan confirming corpus callosum agenesis.

Treatment

- Conservative: parent education. Referral to speech and language therapy, neuropsychologist, neurology and physiotherapy.
- Medical: there is no specific treatment. Manage epilepsy, see pages 146–151.

Complications

- Hydrocephalus.
- Porencephalic cysts.

MAP 13.3 **X-linked Recessive Disorders** (*Continued*)

Complications

- Arrhythmias.
- Epilepsy.
- Gastro-oesophageal reflux disease.
- Osteoporosis.

KLINEFELTER'S SYNDROME

What is Klinefelter's syndrome?

This is a syndrome in which males have an extra X chromosome. Chromosomally, patients are XXY.

Causes

- An additional X chromosome.

Signs and symptoms

- Hypogonadism.
- Long limbs.
- Late onset of puberty.
- Gynaecomastia.
- Infertility.

Investigations

- Prenatal diagnosis.
- Follicle stimulating hormone (FSH) and luteinising hormone (LH) levels.

Treatment

- Conservative: patient and parent education. Genetic counselling.
- Medical: no specific medical therapy. Treat comorbidities such as depression, which is common in this group.

Complications

- Infertility.
- Depression.

Map 13.3 X-linked Recessive Disorders

203   Genetic Disorders

Map 13.4 Autosomal Dominant Conditions

HUNTINGTON'S DISEASE

What is Huntington's disease?

This is an autosomal dominant inherited neurodegenerative disorder.

Causes

- Abnormal *huntingtin* gene on chromosome 4.
- Leads to $(CAG)_n$ repeats.
- The longer the $(CAG)_n$ repeats, the earlier the onset of disease.

Signs and symptoms

- Present at ~35 years of age.
- Progressive decline in motor coordination.
- Chorea.
- Cognitive decline.
- Personality change.

Investigations

- Genetic testing confirms diagnosis.

Treatment

- Conservative: patient education. Genetic counselling.
- Medical: there is no specific treatment. Manage complications.

Complications

- Chorea.
- Dementia.
- Dysphagia.
- Depression.
- Anxiety.

MAP 13.4 **Autosomal Dominant Conditions**

FAMILIAL ADENOMATOUS POLYPOSIS (FAP)

What is FAP?

This is an autosomal dominant condition that causes thousands of polyps to develop in the large intestine. It predisposes patients to colon cancer.

Causes

- Mutation in the *APC* gene on chromosome 5.

Signs and symptoms

- Blood in stool.
- Signs of malignancy, see page 48.

Investigations

See page 48.

- Genetic testing and colonoscopy are diagnostic.

Treatment

- Surgical resection of the affected bowel is the treatment of choice.

Complications

- Colon cancer.

EHLERS–DANLOS SYNDROME

What is Ehlers–Danlos syndrome?

This is a type of connective tissue disorder that results from defective collagen.

Causes

- Defect in type I and type III collagen synthesis.

Signs and symptoms

Remember these as **HBO**:

- **H**yperextension.
- **B**ruise easily.
- **O**steoarthritis (early onset).

Investigations

- Collagen gene mutation testing.
- Skin biopsy for collagen typing.
- ECHO for valvular heart disease and aortic dilation.

Treatment

- Conservative: patient education.
- Medical: there is no specific treatment for this condition. Manage complications.

Complications

- Valvular heart disease.
- Joint deformities, e.g. osteoarthritis and scoliosis.
- Anal prolapse.
- Complications during pregnancy.

Map 13.4 Autosomal Dominant Conditions

Map 13.5 Autosomal Dominant Conditions

MAP 13.5 Autosomal Dominant Conditions (*Continued*)

TUBEROUS SCLEROSIS

What is tuberous sclerosis?

This condition causes nonmalignant tumours to grow in a variety of organs.

Causes

- Mutation of *TSC1* and *TSC2* genes. *TSC1* gene codes for hamartin protein. *TCS2* gene codes for tuberin protein.

Signs and symptoms

These depend on where the tumours form. Some examples include:

- Renal angiomyolipomas: haematuria.
- Rhabdomyomas: cardiac arrhythmias.
- Facial angiofibromas: butterfly distribution on face.
- Ash leaf spots.
- Coloboma.

Investigations

- Fundoscopy.
- Examine skin with Wood's lamp for ash leaf spots and angiofibromas.
- Radiology: CT scan, MRI scan, ECHO (rhabdomyoma), renal ultrasound scan (angiomyolipoma).

MARFAN'S SYNDROME

What is Marfan's syndrome?

This is a disorder of connective tissue due to abnormal fibrillin-1 formation.

Causes

- Mutated *FBN1* gene.

Signs and symptoms

A – **A**rachnodactyly, **A**stigmatism, **A**ngina, **A**ortic **A**neurysm/dissection.

B – **B**ullae, **B**ronchiectasis.

C – **C**yanosis, **C**ysts (spinal), **C**oarctation of the aorta.

D – **D**olichostenomelia, **D**islocation of lens.

P – **P**ectus carinatum/excavatum, high **P**alate, **P**alpitations.

Investigations

- This is a clinical diagnosis.
- ECG and ECHO to monitor cardiac complications.
- MRI scan of spinal cord to monitor neurological complications.

Treatment

- Conservative: patient education.
- Medical: there is no specific treatment. Manage complications.

Complications

- Renal failure.
- Status epilepticus.
- Sudden unexpected death in epilepsy (SUDEP).

Treatment

- Conservative: patient education. Genetic counselling.
- Medical: there is no specific treatment. Manage complications, e.g. prescribe a beta-blocker (if not contraindicated) to reduce blood pressure.
- Surgery: to manage complications.

Complications

- Aortic dissection/aneurysm.
- Valvular disease.
- Glaucoma.
- Scoliosis.
- Depression.

Map 13.5 Autosomal Dominant Conditions

Map 13.6 Autosomal Recessive Conditions

PHENYLKETONURIA

What is phenylketonuria?

This is an autosomal recessive disease in which levels of phenylalanine increase due to the lack of phenylalanine hydroxylase (PAH). Phenylalanine is subsequently converted to phenylpyruvate instead of tyrosine.

Causes
• Mutation in the gene that codes for PAH.

Signs and symptoms
• Asymptomatic at birth.
• Severe learning difficulties.
• Seizures.

Investigations
• Guthrie heel prick test is diagnostic.

Treatment
• Conservative: parent education. Genetic counselling.
• Patients are on lifelong low phenylalanine diet.

Complications
• Neurobehavioural problems.
• Seizures.

MAP 13.6 **Autosomal Recessive Conditions**

FRIEDREICH'S ATAXIA

What is Friedreich's ataxia?

This is an autosomal recessive condition that causes neural degeneration.

Causes
• Mutation of *FXN* gene on chromosome 9 causes GAA repeats and abnormal frataxin production.

Signs and symptoms
• Abnormal gait.
• Speech disturbance.
• Cardiomyopathy.

Investigations
• Genetic testing.
• Nerve conduction studies.
• ECG for cardiac complications.
• Vitamin E levels: rule out vitamin E deficiency as a differential diagnosis.

Treatment
• Conservative: patient and parent education. Refer to physiotherapy and speech and language therapy.
• Medical: there is no specific treatment for this condition. Manage complications.

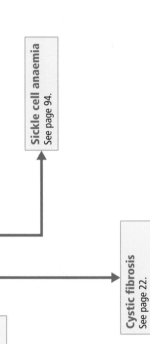

Complications
- Cardiomyopathy.
- Scoliosis.
- Pes cavus (high instep).
- Diabetes mellitus.
- Hearing loss.

Cystic fibrosis
See page 22.

Sickle cell anaemia
See page 94.

Thalassaemia
See page 96.

Map 13.7 Trisomies

MAP 13.7
Trisomies

DOWN'S SYNDROME
What is Down's syndrome?
Down's syndrome is the most common trisomy abnormality, which is characterised by specific signs and symptoms.

Causes
- Trisomy 21.

Signs and symptoms
- Learning difficulties.
- Short stature.
- Flattened nose.
- Slanted eyes.
- Simian crease.
- Gap between 1st and 2nd toe.

Investigations
- Antenatal testing: ultrasound for nuchal translucency.
- Radiology: pelvic X-ray shows dysplastic pelvis.
- ECG and ECHO for cardiac complications.

Treatment
- Conservative: parent education.
- Medical: management of complications.
- Surgical: management of complications.

Complications
- Atrial septal defects.

EDWARD'S SYNDROME
What is Edward's syndrome?
Edward's syndrome is the second most common trisomy abnormality.

Causes
- Trisomy 18.

Signs and symptoms
- Rocker bottom feet.
- Learning difficulties.
- Clenched hands.
- Low set ears.
- Micrognathia.
- Cleft lip or cleft palate.
- Undescended testicles.

Investigations
- Chromosomal analysis confirms diagnosis.
- ECG and ECHO for cardiac complications.

Treatment
- Conservative: parent education and support particularly since life expectancy is 4 months – 1 year.

Complications
- Coarctation of the aorta.
- Atrial septal defects.

- Ventricular septal defects.
- Duodenal atresia.
- Acute lymphoblastic leukaemia.
- Alzheimer's diease.
- Hypothyroidism.

- Inguinal hernia.
- Omphalocoele.
- Renal agenesis.

PATAU'S SYNDROME

What is Patau's syndrome?

This is a chromosomal abnormality.

Causes

- Trisomy 13.

Signs and symptoms

- Learning difficulties.
- Congenital heart disease.
- Cleft lip/palate.
- Microcephaly.
- Polydactyly.
- Rocker bottom feet.

Investigations

- Chromosomal analysis confirms diagnosis.
- ECG and ECHO for cardiac complications.

Treatment

- Conservative: parent education and support particularly since life expectancy is <1 year.

Complications

- Omphalocoele.
- Polycystic kidneys.
- Ventricular septal defects.
- Inguinal hernia.

Table 14.1 Issues in Preterm Infants

TABLE 14.1 Issues in Preterm Infants

Disorder	Comment
Patent ductus arteriosus	Continuous machinery murmur Bounding pulse Treatment: Prostaglandin synthase inhibitor, indomethacin and ibuprofen
Vulnerable to heat loss	Due to: ↓ Subcutaneous fat Heat loss through thin skin Large surface area to volume ratio
Increased infection risk	This is because most IgG is transferred in the last trimester
Necrotising enterocolitis	Bacterial invasion of ischaemic bowel X-ray visualises distended bowel loops due to intramural gas and thickened walls Treat with antibiotics and supportive treatment; may require surgical intervention
Retinopathy of prematurity	Affects blood vessels of the retina and may lead to blindness
Bronchopulmonary dysplasia	CXR shows opacification

TABLE 14.2 Issues in Term Infants

Disorder	Comment
Milk aspiration	↑ Risk with cleft palate
Transient tachypnoea of the newborn	CXR shows fluid in the horizontal fissure
Meconium aspiration	CXR visualises overinflated lungs, areas of consolidation and evidence of collapse

Infection	Common examples:
	• Group B *Streptococcus*
	• Meningitis
	• Conjunctivitis:
	   ○ Group B *Streptococcus*
	   ○ *Listeria monocytogenes*
	   ○ *Escherichia coli*
	• Hepatitis B

Persistent pulmonary hypertension of the newborn	This condition is life threatening Treat with nitric oxide inhalation and sildenafil

Map 14.1 Hernias

What is a hernia?

A hernia is the protrusion of a viscus or part of a viscus through a weakening in its containing cavity.

There are many different types of hernia, e.g.:

- Inguinal hernia.
- Femoral hernia.
- Hiatus hernia.
- Umbilical hernia: this is a hernia that is more common in males and is due to weakness of the umbilicus. It is usually self-resolving.
- Incisional hernia: weakness caused by a surgical repair that has not fully healed.

INGUINAL

Types

There are two types of inguinal hernia:

- Direct:
  - Causes: due to weakness in the abdominal wall.
  - Located **medial** to the inferior epigastric vessels.
- Indirect:
  - Causes: due to a congenital weakness of the internal inguinal ring.
  - Located **lateral** to the inferior epigastric vessels.
  - More common than direct hernias.

Signs and symptoms

- Mass in the groin.
- Hernia accentuated by certain situations such as coughing or on standing.
- Reducible.
- Pain: hernia likely to be strangulated, i.e. the blood supply is compromised.

Investigations

- This is a clinical diagnosis.
- Radiology: ultrasound scan of hernia.

Treatment

- Surgical hernia repair is the treatment of choice.

Complications

- Strangulation.
- Incarceration.

MAP 14.1 **Hernias**

HIATUS

Types
There are two types of hiatus hernia: sliding and rolling.

Causes
Weakness in the diaphragm that allows the stomach and intestines to move into the chest cavity. There are certain risk factors that make this more likely, e.g. obesity and constipation.

Signs and symptoms
- Those of gastro-oesophageal reflux disease (GORD), see page 42.

Investigations
- Endoscopy.
- Barium study.

Treatment
- Those of GORD, see page 42.

Complications
- Strangulation.
- Gastric volvulus.
- Those of GORD, see page 42.

FEMORAL

Causes
Due to a weakness in the femoral canal.
- Located inferior and lateral to the pubic tubercle.
- More common in females.
- High risk of strangulation.

Signs and symptoms
- Mass in the groin.
- Tends to be irreducible.

Investigations
- This is a clinical diagnosis.
- Radiology: ultrasound scan of hernia.

Treatment
- Surgical hernia repair is the treatment of choice.

Complications
- Strangulation.
- Fistula formation.

Map 14.1 Hernias

Map 14.2 Glaucoma

What is glaucoma?

Glaucoma is a group of eye disorders that are characterised by visual field loss, alterations to the optic disc and damage to the optic nerve. Intraocular pressure (IOP) is usually increased but it may, in some cases, be normal.

Open angle

- Causes: *MYOC* mutation. A secondary cause is obstruction of the trabecular meshwork by trauma.
- Most common.
- ↑ IOP.
- Painless.

Closed angle

- Causes: may be split into primary and secondary causes:
  ○ Primary causes: shallow anterior chambers.
  ○ Secondary causes: trauma and tumours of the ciliary body.
- This is a medical emergency.
- Peripheral zone of iris adheres to the trabecular meshwork.
- ↑ IOP since aqueous outflow is impeded.
- Painful.

Treatment

- Conservative: patient education. Annual screening.
- Medical:
  ○ Prostaglandin analogues, e.g. latanoprost:
    – mode of action (MOA): ↑ uveoscleral outflow of aqueous humour.
  ○ Beta-receptor antagonists, e.g. betaxolol:
    – MOA: ↓ aqueous humour production.
  ○ Alpha-2 agonists, e.g. brimonidine:
    – MOA: ↓ aqueous humour production and ↑ uveoscleral outflow of aqueous humour.
  ○ Less selective alpha agonists, e.g. adrenaline:
    – MOA: ↓ aqueous humour production.
    – Do not use in closed angle glaucoma.
  ○ Miotic agents (parasympathomimetics), e.g. pilocarpine:
    – MOA: ↑ uveoscleral outflow of aqueous humour by causing the ciliary muscles to contract and open the trabecular meshwork.
  ○ Carbonic anhydrase inhibitors, e.g. dorzolamide:
    – MOA: ↓ aqueous humour secretion by inhibiting carbonic anhydrase in the ciliary body.
  ○ Cholinesterase inhibitors, e.g. physostigmine.

MAP 14.2 **Glaucoma**

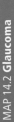

Characteristics

Remember **VIA:**

- **V**isual field changes due to peripheral field loss.
- ↑ **I**OP.
- **A**lterations to the optic nerve cup.

Investigations

- Tonometry: measures IOP.
- Fundoscopy.
- Visual field test: tunnel vision is a late feature.
- Gonioscopy: assesses the iridocorneal angle.
- Scanning laser ophthalmoscopy.
- Scanning laser polarimetry.

Complications

- Blindness.

Map 14.2 Glaucoma

Map 14.3 Hearing Loss

SENSORINEURAL

What is sensorineural hearing loss?

This is hearing loss that occurs due to a problem within the inner ear or involving the vestibulocochlear nerve.

Causes

- Congenital:
  - ○ Rubella.
  - ○ Genetic causes, e.g. Alport's syndrome.
- Acquired:
  - ○ Noise injury.
  - ○ Head injury.
  - ○ Infection, e.g. meningitis, measles, mumps, syphilis.
  - ○ Presbycusis.
  - ○ Tumour, e.g. acoustic neuroma.
  - ○ Ototoxic drugs, e.g. aminoglycosides, furosemide.
  - ○ Ménière's disease.

Treatment

- Conservative: patient and parent education. Advise about sign language programmes if appropriate. Hearing aids (if these are not suitable or do not work then consider middle ear and cochlear implants).
- Medical: antivirals, antifungals or antibiotics if indicated.

Investigations

- Bloods: look for underlying cause if indicated.
- Audiometric hearing test.
- Weber test.
- Rinne test.

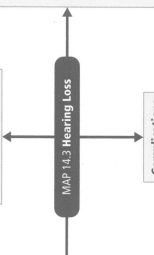

MAP 14.3 **Hearing Loss**

Complications

- Depression.
- Anxiety.

CONDUCTIVE

What is conductive hearing loss?

This is hearing loss that occurs due to abnormalities/blockage of the middle ear or of the auditory canal. It may be reversible.

Causes

- Congenital:
  - ○ Abnormalities of the ossicles.
  - ○ Ear atresia.
  - ○ Complications of Down's syndrome and Pierre Robin sequence.
- Acquired:
  - ○ Wax.
  - ○ Otitis externa.
  - ○ Glue ear.
  - ○ Perforated drum.
  - ○ Otosclerosis.
  - ○ Eustachian tube dysfunction.

Treatment

- Treatment of underlying cause.

Name of criteria	Name of disease
Framingham Criteria	Congestive cardiac failure
New York Heart Association Classification	Heart failure
Duke Criteria	Infective endocarditis
The Los Angeles Classification	Gastro-oesophageal reflux disease
The Rome III Criteria	Irritable bowel syndrome
The Rockall Risk Scoring Criteria	Upper gastrointestinal bleeding
The Child–Pugh Grading System	Cirrhosis and risk of variceal bleeding
The Truelove and Witts Criteria	Ulcerative colitis
The Vienna Criteria	Crohn's disease
The Rifle Criteria	Acute kidney injury
MRC Classification	Grading for muscle power
The McDonald Criteria	Multiple sclerosis
Duke's Criteria	Colorectal cancer
Ann Arbor Staging	Hodgkin and non-Hodgkin lymphoma
Beighton Criteria	Joint hypermobility
Psoriasis Area and Severity Index	Psoriasis
Cardiac Failure, Hypertension, Age, Diabetes, Stroke system (CHADS2) Score	Calculates risk of stroke in patients with AF
QRISK Score	Calculates 10-year cardiovascular risk

Disease	Page No.	Website
Heart failure	4	http://www.nice.org.uk/nicemedia/live/13099/50526/50526.pdf
Myocardial infarction	6	MI with STEMI: http://www.nice.org.uk/nicemedia/live/14208/64410/64410.pdf Unstable angina and NSTEMI: http://www.nice.org.uk/nicemedia/live/12949/47924/47924.pdf Secondary prevention: http://www.nice.org.uk/nicemedia/pdf/CG48NICEGuidance.pdf
Angina pectoris	8	http://guidance.nice.org.uk/nicemedia/live/13549/55663/55663.pdf
Infective endocarditis	10	Prophylaxis against infective endocarditis: http://www.nice.org.uk/nicemedia/pdf/CG64NICEguidance.pdf Guidelines on the prevention, diagnosis, and treatment of infective endocarditis: http://eurheartj.oxfordjournals.org/content/30/19/2369.full.pdf
Hypertension	16	http://www.nice.org.uk/nicemedia/live/13561/56015/56015.pdf http://www.nice.org.uk/nicemedia/live/13561/56008/56008.pdf
Atrial fibrillation	18	http://www.nice.org.uk/nicemedia/live/10982/30054/30054.pdf Full guideline: http://www.nice.org.uk/nicemedia/live/10982/30055/30055.pdf https://cardiology.ucsf.edu/care/clinical/electro/fib-management.html
Pneumonia	20	https://www.brit-thoracic.org.uk/Portals/0/Guidelines/Pneumonia/CAPQuickRefGuide-web.pdf
Bronchiectasis	22	https://www.brit-thoracic.org.uk/document-library/clinical-information/bronchiectasis/bts-guideline-for-non-cf-bronchiectasis/
Asthma	24	https://www.brit-thoracic.org.uk/document-library/clinical-information/asthma/btssign-asthma-guideline-quick-reference-guide/ Full guideline: https://www.brit-thoracic.org.uk/document-library/clinical-information/asthma/btssign-guideline-on-the-management-of-asthma/
Chronic obstructive pulmonary disease	26	http://www.nice.org.uk/nicemedia/live/13029/49399/49399.pdf Full guideline: http://www.nice.org.uk/nicemedia/live/13029/49425/49425.pdf

Continued on next page

223

Continued from previous page

Disease	Page No.	Website
Lung cancer	30	http://www.nice.org.uk/nicemedia/live/13465/54202/54202.pdf
Deep vein thrombosis	31	Including Wells score: http://www.nice.org.uk/nicemedia/live/13767/59720/59720.pdf
Pulmonary embolism	32	http://www.nice.org.uk/nicemedia/live/13767/59720/59720.pdf http://www.ncbi.nlm.nih.gov/pmc/articles/PMC1746692/pdf/v058p00470.pdf
Pneumothorax	34	https://www.brit-thoracic.org.uk/document-library/clinical-information/pleural-disease/pleural-disease-guidelines-2010/pleural-disease-guideline-quick-reference-guide/
Upper GI bleeding	37	http://www.nice.org.uk/nicemedia/live/13762/59549/59549.pdf
Irritable bowel syndrome	38	http://www.nice.org.uk/nicemedia/live/11927/39622/39622.pdf
Ulcerative colitis	40	http://www.nice.org.uk/nicemedia/live/14189/64216/64216.pdf
Crohn's disease	40	http://www.nice.org.uk/nicemedia/live/13936/61001/61001.pdf
Hepatitis B	46	http://www.nice.org.uk/nicemedia/live/14191/64234/64234.pdf
Colorectal cancer	48	http://www.nice.org.uk/nicemedia/live/13597/56998/56998.pdf Full guideline: http://www.nice.org.uk/nicemedia/live/13597/56957/56957.pdf
Acute pancreatitis	50	http://www.bsg.org.uk/images/stories/docs/clinical/guidelines/pancreatic/pancreatic.pdf
Urinary tract infection	58	http://www.sign.ac.uk/pdf/sign88.pdf
Acute kidney injury	62	http://www.nice.org.uk/nicemedia/live/14258/65056/65056.pdf
Chronic kidney injury	62	http://www.nice.org.uk/nicemedia/live/12069/42117/42117.pdf
Hypothyroidism and hyperthyroidism	72, 74	http://www.btf-thyroid.org/images/stories/pdf/tft_guideline_final_version_july_2006.pdf
Thyroid cancer	76	http://www.btf-thyroid.org/images/stories/pdf/thyroid_cancer_guidelines_2007.pdf
Diabetes mellitus	78	Type 1: http://www.nice.org.uk/nicemedia/live/10944/29393/29393.pdf http://www.nice.org.uk/nicemedia/live/10944/29396/29396.pdf Type 2: http://www.nice.org.uk/nicemedia/live/12165/44320/44320.pdf

Disease	Page No.	Website
Cushing's syndrome	88	https://www.endocrine.org/~/media/endosociety/Files/Publications/Clinical%20Practice%20Guidelines/Cushings_Guideline.pdf
Anaemia	94	http://www.momentum.nhs.uk/pathology/Haematology/Guidelines%20on%20anaemia.htm
		Iron deficiency anaemia: http://www.bsg.org.uk/pdf_word_docs/iron_def.pdf
Malaria	106	http://www.hpa.org.uk/webc/HPAwebFile/HPAweb_C/1194947343507
Tuberculosis	108	http://www.nice.org.uk/nicemedia/live/13422/53642/53642.pdf
HIV	112	http://www.who.int/hiv/pub/guidelines/en/
Stroke	140	http://www.nice.org.uk/nicemedia/live/12018/41331/41331.pdf
Dementia	142	http://sign.ac.uk/pdf/sign86.pdf
Epilepsy	146	http://www.nice.org.uk/nicemedia/live/13635/57779/57779.pdf
Parkinson's disease	152	http://www.nice.org.uk/nicemedia/live/10984/30088/30088.pdf
Multiple sclerosis	153	http://www.nice.org.uk/nicemedia/live/10930/29199/29199.pdf
Rheumatoid arthritis	157	http://www.nice.org.uk/nicemedia/live/12131/43329/43329.pdf
		Full guideline: http://www.nice.org.uk/nicemedia/live/12131/43326/43326.pdf
Osteoarthritis	157	http://www.nice.org.uk/nicemedia/live/14383/66527/66527.pdf
		http://www.webmd.com/osteoporosis/living-with-osteoporosis-7/tests
Psoriasis	160	http://www.nice.org.uk/nicemedia/live/13938/61190/61190.pdf
		http://www.sign.ac.uk/pdf/sign121.pdf
Psoriatic arthritis	160	http://www.sign.ac.uk/pdf/sign121.pdf
		http://www.nice.org.uk/nicemedia/live/13110/50422/50422.pdf
Osteoporosis	166	Primary prevention: http://www.nice.org.uk/nicemedia/live/11746/47176/47176.pdf
		Secondary prevention: http://www.nice.org.uk/nicemedia/live/11748/42447/42447.pdf
Mastitis	178	http://www.nice.org.uk/nicemedia/pdf/CG37NICEguideline.pdf

Continued on next page

Continued from previous page

Disease	Page No.	Website
Breast cancer	180	Advanced: http://www.nice.org.uk/nicemedia/live/11778/43308/43308.pdf Early and locally advanced: http://www.nice.org.uk/nicemedia/live/12132/43314/43314.pdf Referral for suspected cancer: http://www.nice.org.uk/nicemedia/live/10968/29814/29814.pdf
Glaucoma	218	http://www.nice.org.uk/nicemedia/live/12145/43839/43839.pdf

Index

Index